P9-DCZ-157
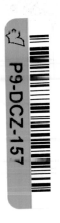

Fitness and Nutrition

Also in the Growing, Growing Strong:
A Whole Health Curriculum for Young Children Series

Body Care

Safety

Social and Emotional Well-Being

Community and Environment

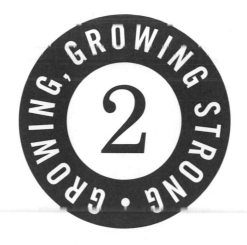

GROWING, GROWING STRONG

2

A Whole Health Curriculum for Young Children

Fitness and Nutrition

Third Edition

Connie Jo Smith
Charlotte M. Hendricks
Becky S. Bennett

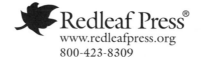

Redleaf Press®
www.redleafpress.org
800-423-8309

Published by Redleaf Press
10 Yorkton Court
St. Paul, MN 55117
www.redleafpress.org

© 1997, 2006, 2014 by Connie Jo Smith, Charlotte M. Hendricks, and Becky S. Bennett

All rights reserved. Unless otherwise noted on a specific page, no portion of this publication may be reproduced or transmitted in any form or by any means, electronic or mechanical, including photocopying, recording, or capturing on any information storage and retrieval system, without permission in writing from the publisher, except by a reviewer, who may quote brief passages in a critical article or review to be printed in a magazine or newspaper, or electronically transmitted on radio, television, or the Internet.

First edition published 1997. Second edition 2006. Third edition 2014.
Cover design by Jim Handrigan
Cover photograph by Blend Images Photography/Veer
Interior design by Percolator
Typeset in Stone Informal, Matrix Script, and Trade Gothic
Illustrations by Chris Wold Dyrud
Photograph on page 83 © Wavebreakmediamicrro/Veer
Printed in the United States of America
20 19 18 17 16 15 14 13   1 2 3 4 5 6 7 8

Library of Congress Cataloging-in-Publication Data
Smith, Connie Jo.
    Fitness and nutrition / Connie Jo Smith, Charlotte M. Hendricks, Becky S. Bennett. — Third edition.
      pages cm. — (Growing, growing strong : a whole health curriculum for young children)
    Summary: "Given the recent rise of childhood obesity, the need for health education is needed more than ever. This curriculum provides developmentally appropriate activities that introduce important health concepts, including physical activity, rest and relaxation, and nutrition and eating habits."— Provided by publisher.
    ISBN 978-1-60554-241-6 (pbk.)
    ISBN 978-1-60554-332-1 (e-book)
    1. Health education (Preschool)—United States. 2. Health education (Elementary)—United States.
    3. Curriculum planning—United States.   I. Hendricks, Charlotte M., 1957- II. Bennett, Becky S., 1954- III. Title.
    LB1140.5.H4S647 2013
    372.37—dc23
                                                                                                                2013019776

CHILDREN'S DEPARTMENT
Falmouth Public Library
300 Main Street
Falmouth, MA 02540

Printed on acid-free paper

To the memory of my parents, Nevolyn and George. My mother taught me that a sense of humor is an essential life skill, regardless of age. My dad taught me the importance of love and independence.

—Connie Jo

To Gayle Cunningham for guidance and friendship, and to Don Palmer for always being there for me. And in memory of Nic Frising for showing the humor in life through art.

—Charlotte

To the memory of my parents, Charlie and Jeanette, who gave me life, love, and encouragement to follow my dreams. And to my partner, Connie, who has taught me so much about the early care and education field, love, and family.

—Becky

Contents

Acknowledgments

We would like to express heartfelt appreciation to our talented, hardworking, and ever-positive editor, Kyra Ostendorf. This book is much richer for her ideas, guidance, and smiles—those given in person and those that arrived through electronic communication ;-). Thanks to Elena Fultz and Grace Fowler, interns at Redleaf Press, who assisted in technical editing. We are grateful to David Heath for his initial editing support and encouragement. And, of course, we want to acknowledge all the individuals we have had professional encounters with over the years, as each contact has helped us grow and has enhanced our work.

Introduction

Children have many new and exciting experiences during their preschool and childhood years. They meet new people and make friends, explore their environment, and begin to learn new skills. Many lifelong habits begin during the early childhood years, including behaviors that can affect health and physical development. By encouraging healthy eating and regular physical activity, teachers can promote healthy weight and prevention of childhood obesity.

Early childhood is a time for new experiences with food. New foods are introduced at home, at schools, at restaurants, and at the homes of friends and relatives, and familiar foods are sometimes prepared in unfamiliar ways. For example, a child who recognizes chicken in the form of chicken fingers may be surprised to see a whole raw chicken or even a live chicken! Chicken may be fried, baked, grilled, or stewed. Likewise, fruits may be fresh, canned, frozen, or dried. Vegetables can be served raw, stir-fried, sautéed, baked, boiled, grilled, or fried.

Children explore food with all their senses. First, they see and smell the food. Fresh produce provides a rainbow of colors: red strawberries, green broccoli, and yellow squash, for example. The smell of a grilling hamburger or baking cookies may entice children to run and see what is cooking. Adding to the sensory experience, children then hear the sounds produced by the food, such as crackers breaking, fish sizzling, and apples crunching. Next, young children explore the food's texture and temperature, first with their fingers and then with their lips and tongues. Finally, children taste the food and discover whether it is sweet, sour, salty, or spicy. Through exploration and play, children learn about the variety of foods available and begin to make food choices.

Many lifelong eating habits, including food likes and dislikes, are shaped during the early years of childhood. Young children will not know and do not need to understand which nutrients are in specific foods. Nor do they need to know how many grams of fat are in their lunches. They do need to develop an appreciation for the wide variety of foods available. By eating foods in a variety of colors, textures, temperatures, and tastes, most children will consume the nutrients they need for healthful growth and development.

The adult's role in children's nutrition is to provide nutritionally balanced meals and snacks. Foods that are appealing and interesting to children are the

1

most likely to be eaten. Be aware that some children may not want to taste or even touch an unfamiliar food. Continue to offer nutritious foods, and consider preparing them in various ways and involving children through classroom food activities. Children who do not want an unfamiliar or undesirable food on their plates may be receptive to receiving very small amounts of the food on small side plates. Numerous exposures to a food may be necessary before children decide whether they like or dislike the food.

In addition to having new experiences with food, young children have new experiences as they move their bodies and engage in physical activity. Three- and four-year-olds are developing basic gross-motor skills, like running and jumping. Fine-motor skills are developing as children grasp large items and fat crayons and progress to grasping smaller manipulatives and then printing. Gaining control of body movements and developing specific physical skills do not occur just as children grow older. Physical skill requires demonstration, exploration of possibilities, and practice.

Most children enjoy active physical play, and regular physical activity is essential to healthful growth and development. Both indoor and outdoor physical activities allow children to interact with others, explore, and learn. By providing safe environments, encouraging exploration, and challenging children to try new movements, you can help children build a foundation for healthy, active lives.

Topics in this curriculum include motor development, fitness and physical activity, rest and relaxation, food choices and eating habits, and avoidance of germs when eating. The activities and resources will help children become aware of their bodies. Children will learn about different body parts and how they work together, differences in body shape and size, and how to take care of their bodies. This knowledge will help children be proud of their bodies.

Each chapter covers one topic and starts with an overview that includes suggested interest area materials, learning objectives, vocabulary words to introduce and use (which should include vocabulary words in the languages spoken by the families of children in the class), supports for creating the learning environment, and suggestions for evaluating children's understanding of the topic. The overview is followed by activity ideas. Icons appear with each activity to identify the areas of development and learning integrated into the activity:

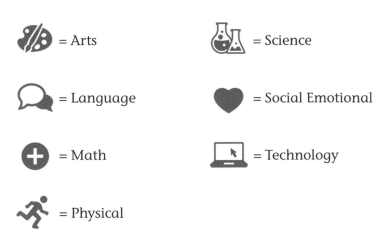

= Arts   = Science

= Language   = Social Emotional

= Math   = Technology

= Physical

Each chapter concludes with a family information page and a take-home family activity page, both of which can be photocopied from the book and distributed to families. These pages can also be downloaded from the Growing, Growing Strong page at www.redleafpress.org for electronic sharing.

INTEREST AREA MATERIALS

Dramatic Play

multiethnic dolls and toy people with body parts that move and bend

dream catchers

yoga mats

sleepwear and robes

pillows and cushions

chef hats

pot holders

aprons

sleeping bags

exercise clothes

empty, clean food containers

centerpieces

tablecloths

cloth napkins and napkin rings

spice containers

edible herbs, such as mint and lemongrass

tongs

serving spoons

green beans to string and snap

notepads

writing tools

Blocks

catalogs of kitchen cabinets and furniture

toy food to haul

toy pots and pans for hauling

large seeds to haul, including clean peach pits and avocado seeds

clean, empty food boxes for building

clean, empty food cans for building (Cover sharp edges with heavy tape.)

clean, empty milk and juice containers for building

artificial aquarium plants for landscaping

pictures of restaurants and groceries

napkin rings for hauling and building

paper cups for building

Table Toys

food and plant puzzles

exercise- and sports-related puzzles

toy fruit to sort and match to pictures

lotto and domino games that feature food

tongs, trays, and objects to manipulate

wind-up toys

Art

food magazines	still life centerpieces
glow-in-the-dark paint	garbage bag ties
kits for making pot holders	chenille stems
straws	vinyl-coated wire
pottery clay	yarn
nontoxic berries for making dye	

Language Arts

food container labels	seed catalogs
exercise equipment advertisements	restaurant menus
cookbooks	physical fitness charts
recipes	pictures of people exercising
blank recipe cards	pictures of people playing sports
gardening magazines	chalkboard and chalk or chart paper and markers for writing menus

Library

The Napping House by Audrey Wood

The Greedy Python by Richard Buckley

The Empanadas That Abuela Made/Las empandas que hacía la abuela by Diane Gonzales Bertrand

Kitten's First Full Moon by Kevin Henkes

Science and Math

stopwatches	foods to weigh, such as various sizes of apples or potatoes
lava lamps	potted plants or a garden (Radishes and leaf lettuce grow quickly in cool climates. Basil, dill, mint, and parsley grow quickly in most climates.)
aquarium	
seed packets to sort	
dry beans to sort	
pictures of the digestive system	spices to taste
raw food—such as potato peels or raw potato, bread, or apple slices—for handling and observing change	napkin rings to count and sort
	night-lights to examine
scales	music boxes

Outdoors

hammock	balls of many sizes
tent	scarves
watercooler and cups	hoops
picnic table or plastic tablecloth	streamers
shovels	stopwatches
rakes	toy airplanes to fly
containers for collecting seeds	kites to fly
disconnected sections of water hoses	portable music player for dancing
jump ropes	whistles

Technology

exercise videos	flashlights
sports videos	massagers
dance videos	sleep sound machines or sleep sound applications on a multi-touch mobile device
cooking show videos	
software, applications, or websites showing digestion	see-through music boxes
	wind-up radios with hand cranks

Sand, Water, and Construction

hourglass sand timers for measuring exercise time	obstacle course materials for constructing courses and mazes
wave machine to watch and replicate	
sand pit for running and broad jumping	

Watch Me Move My Body!

LEARNING OBJECTIVES

- Children will demonstrate specific body movements (for example, lifting their legs or waving their arms).
- Children will recognize body parts associated with specific movements (for example, fingers for wiggling and arms and hands for throwing a ball).
- Children will recognize and show acceptance of different physical abilities.

Physical development and movement skills are the foundation for much of what young children do throughout the day. Movement helps children develop physically, cognitively, and emotionally; children move to learn and learn to move.

Children grow and develop at their own individual rates. Children vary in height, weight, and motor development. During the preschool years, children's body proportions change, and children begin to develop a greater sense of balance and more control of large-muscle movements, such as running, jumping, and climbing. Fine-motor development also develops more fully during the early years as children begin to throw and catch balls, hold crayons, and manipulate small objects.

The development of movement skills is sequential, starting with the head, moving down to the feet, and then progressing from the center of the body to the extremities. Of the extremities, children develop movement coordination with their arms and hands first and then their legs and feet. Physical movement skills further develop as children grow older and practice. Instruction and practice are essential for children to further develop their movement skills. For example, four-year-old children often run with their feet flat on the ground. As they grow older and develop movement skills, their legs and feet become better coordinated, and they begin to run more rhythmically on the balls of their feet.

VOCABULARY

balance	fast	outside	spin
bend	gallop	right	tumble
bounce	inside	roll	up
center	left	round	yoga
collision	maze	skeleton	
crawl	movement	slide	
down	obstacle	slow	

CREATING THE ENVIRONMENT

■ Designate play spaces, both indoors and outdoors, that are large enough to accommodate all the children so they have freedom of movement. Areas should be obstacle-free to prevent tripping. Inspect your play area daily, and remove debris or other potential hazards (for example, stinging insects).

■ Provide a variety of materials and toys (for example, balls, scarves, hoops, and steps) that facilitate a range of movements.

EVALUATION

■ Do children use familiar movements (for example, wiggling fingers or waving arms) in creative ways when demonstrated?

■ Do children try variations of body movements (for example, a big wave of the whole arm or a small wave of the hand)?

■ Do children move specific body parts when instructed (for example, when doing the "Hokey Pokey")?

■ Do children identify specific movements and skills (for example, jumping, running, and skipping) that they do well or are improving?

■ Do children encourage one another when performing or trying movements?

CHILDREN'S ACTIVITIES

Bodies in Motion

Create a ten-minute video showing people (and animals) in motion. Include children in the class, family members, other children and adults in the program, and strangers (with permission). Make sure the video represents a diverse population, including both males and females of different ages, ethnicities, and levels of mobility. Movement ideas include crawling, walking, sliding, running, biking, skiing, hang gliding, skating (roller, ice-, or in-line), golfing, swimming, weight lifting, dancing, exercising, washing a car, playing ball, practicing yoga, hopping, jumping, rocking, bending, climbing, horseback riding, hiking, climbing stairs, moving in a wheelchair, and walking with a walker.

Show the video to children. Encourage them to talk about who they saw, what parts of the body they saw being moved, and what kinds of movement they noticed. Point out to children that people who look different from one another (for example, in gender, ethnicity, age, length of hair, color of skin, and so on) can participate successfully in physical activity. Ask them how they think the people in the video feel as they get ready to move, as they are moving, and after they move. Introduce words that describe the movements. Write down the words so children can see them. Explain that moving our bodies helps us grow strong and stay healthy.

MATERIALS
- a video camera, a viewing device for the video, a whiteboard or chart paper, and markers

OTHER IDEAS

- Arrange a trip to a community gym so children can see people working out, or visit a physical education class at a local school.
  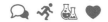

- Visit a sports team during practice so children can interview the players about why they play, what body parts they move during practice, and how they stay fit.

- Visit a gymnastics or dance class or attend a dance recital, or invite a gymnastics or dance teacher to the classroom to demonstrate some ways they move their bodies.

- Visit a cheerleading squad, dance team, color guard, or flag team during practice. Ask members what body parts they exercise.

Bounce and Balance

Create a bouncing experience for children by setting up a variety of bouncing equipment. As children bounce, help them measure how high they are bouncing. Encourage them to express how they feel while they are bouncing and after they stop bouncing.

MATERIALS

- various types of bouncing equipment (such as inner tubes, playground equipment with springs, an air mattress, a large bouncing ball with a handle, or a minitrampoline)

- ❗ Safety Note: Do not use large trampolines. Limit participation so you can closely supervise all bouncing activities. Allow only one child on the equipment at a time. Ask extra adults to supervise and spot children. Reinforce proper safety by using appropriate safety equipment. Check recall notices prior to use of trampolines.

OTHER IDEAS

- Show children objects, and have them guess which ones will bounce. Let them try to balance the objects on their feet, stomachs, hands, and heads while lying down and standing up. When objects fall off, help children measure how high they bounce. Introduce the word *collision,* and explain that a collision occurs when something bounces. As follow-up, look for and discuss other collisions.

- Encourage children to raise one leg and balance on the other. Then ask them to return the lifted leg to the ground and raise the opposite leg, balancing on the other side. Repeat the activity, but ask children to hop up and down on the balancing leg while the other is raised.

- Use any combination of the following materials to create an obstacle course inside or outside: a flat rope to create a curved path; long, narrow boards to create a straight path; large, sturdy building blocks and/or clean tires end to end to form a long, low, raised surface. Have children take turns crawling, walking, and hopping across the surface without falling off.

❶ Safety Note: Be aware that rubber tires contain volatile organic compounds (VOCs) and may also contain heavy metals—do not use tires that are deteriorating.

■ Visit a circus or acrobatic club to observe bouncing, tumbling, and balancing movements.

Let's Bend

In small groups, provide children with bendable art supplies. Invite them to explore the materials. Ask children how the materials are alike. If they do not use the word *bend,* introduce the term and ask them to show you what parts of their bodies they can bend. Ask questions to help them identify bending parts, such as their necks, elbows, knees, ankles, wrists, fingers, toes, and waists. Encourage them to demonstrate the many ways they can bend each body part they name, and then suggest they use the bendable art supplies to mimic bending various body parts.

MATERIALS

- bendable art supplies (such as garbage bag ties, chenille stems, vinyl-coated wire, yarn, plastic lacing, and Wikki Stix)

OTHER IDEAS

- Show children a model or picture of a skeleton, and let them find the places that bend.

- Provide art supplies, and assist children in "bending" paper to make origami creations. The Activity Village website found at www.activityvillage .co.uk provides downloadable instructions, pictures, and videos for creating origami.

- Invite a yoga instructor to visit the classroom and give a yoga demonstration.

- Visit a dance or tae kwon do class, or invite a dance or karate teacher to the classroom to give a demonstration.

Around and Around

Show children a spinning top, and ask them how they think it works. Let them play with several tops. Ask children to move like the top and describe the sensation. Give children hula hoops, streamers, and other materials for making circular motions outside.

MATERIALS

- spinning tops, hula hoops, and streamers

OTHER IDEAS

- Visit an amusement park or carousel to see and feel the movement of the rides.

- Distribute clean tires across an indoor or outdoor open area, and encourage each child to walk around the top of each tire.

- Safety Note: Be aware that rubber tires contain volatile organic compounds (VOCs) and may also contain heavy metals—do not use tires that are deteriorating.

- Have children hold hands and form a circle. Play music, chant, or sing while having children move to the right, then to the left, then to the center, and then out again.

  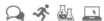

- Play the song "The Bungee Jumpers" by Sharon Shannon or "See Me Spinning" by Lora L. Holmes and Jessie L. Gaynor, and encourage children to move to the music according to the lyrics (jumping or spinning).

  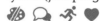

How Many Ways Can You Move?

Gather children in a spacious area, and ask them to show you how many ways they can move. Encourage them to find additional ways to move by watching one another and thinking of animals or machines that move. After a few minutes of moving, ask them to move fast, slow, with someone else, using a prop, without using their feet, with their eyes closed, in a circle, and up and down.

Ask children if they would like to invite their families to see the many ways they have learned to move. If children are interested, form committees and involve them in planning the event. Children may work on creating invitations, finding a location, greeting families, setting up the seating area, choosing music and decorations, and deciding how to tell families what they know about movement and how it makes them feel. Encourage children to think ahead about ways they can move and props they may want to use during the event. In order to keep the event spontaneous and stress-free, do not spend time practicing staged movements. Encourage children to think of ways to involve families in the spontaneous movement. Invite local media to attend the "Moving My Body" show.

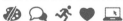

MATERIALS

■ props, decorations, and other materials identified by children

OTHER IDEAS

■ Play the song "I Like to Walk" by Grenadilla, and listen to the words. Let children predict the movements they will see on a walk. Then take them for a walk to observe movements.

■ Create an obstacle course or maze for children inside the classroom or outdoors.

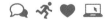

■ Visit a warehouse to see items being moved with equipment, or watch a video clip of equipment that is moving objects.

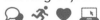

■ Introduce an ant farm to the classroom, and encourage children to watch and describe the ants' movement, activity, and community.

Marbles for Giants

On a floor or flat outdoor surface, outline a large circle with chalk, string, or tape. Place several beach balls (five to ten) within the circle. From outside the circle, use an additional beach ball as the "shooter," allowing children to take turns rolling (or throwing) the shooter in the direction of any of the beach balls within the circle. The goal of the game is to knock beach balls from inside the circle to outside the circle with the shooter. When a beach ball is knocked out of the circle with the shooter, it is considered out of play. Retrieve the shooter, and give it to the next person. Repeat the process until all beach balls have been knocked outside the circle. Increase the difficulty of the game by filling beach balls with water or sand. As another option, number the beach balls inside the circle, and encourage children to knock the beach balls out of the circle in numerical order.

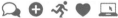

MATERIALS

- several medium to large beach balls; string, tape, or chalk; and markers

OTHER IDEAS

- Play the game Marbles for Giants, but have children in the circle rather than beach balls. Have children sit or stand inside the marked circle on the floor. Allow children to take turns rolling the shooter beach ball from outside the circle to inside the circle, with the goal of gently touching someone who is sitting or standing inside the circle. The child who is touched by the shooter becomes the next person to roll the shooter, trying to touch another person inside the circle.

- Play the game Bowling for Giants by using milk cartons or jugs as bowling pins and beach balls as bowling balls. As an alternative, number the pins, and have children try to knock down pins in numerical order.

- Choose and number stationary items on the playground (for example, posts, signs, and building corners). Make sure the stationary items are isolated and not in the path of playground equipment. With masking tape or rope, mark specific distances on the ground out from each item (to increase or decrease difficulty).

Have children stand on a mark and then roll a beach ball to try to strike the item from varying distances. Then have children move to the next numbered or marked item on the playground.

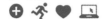

■ Visit a soccer team's practice, and encourage children to talk with the players about how they learned to use their feet and heads to move the ball around the field. Encourage children to ask players questions about what they do and eat to stay in good physical shape.

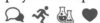

FAMILY INFORMATION

WATCH ME MOVE MY BODY!

Children grow and develop at different rates. Some children are tall or short for their age. Some children seem thin, and some seem stout. Differences are normal and part of growing up, but if you are concerned about your child's physical development, talk with your child's doctor.

Children also develop movement skills at different rates. As children's body proportions change, they begin to develop a greater sense of balance. They also gain more control of their large-muscle movements, such as those used in running, jumping, and climbing. Differences in rates of development are normal. For example, a few children may be able to ride a two-wheel bicycle at age three, but most children will not develop this skill until age five, six, or even older!

Children do not develop movement skills just from growing older. Movement and physical skill development takes time, instruction, and lots of practice.

ENCOURAGE ACTIVE PLAY

Play with your child, and offer encouragement as he or she practices new movement skills. Learning a new movement begins when your child sees the movement demonstrated by you or other children. New movements might include throwing a ball, jumping rope, or climbing the ladder on the slide. As your child tries new movements, support her or his efforts, and challenge her or him to explore ways to be successful. Your budding ball player may start by rolling a ball and tossing it underhand before trying to throw an overhand pitch. Start slow and easy, and offer lots of praise and encouragement! Encourage your child to run, play, and be active whenever possible—both indoors and outdoors.

From *Fitness and Nutrition* by Connie Jo Smith, Charlotte M. Hendricks, and Becky S. Bennett, © 2014. Published by Redleaf Press, www.redleafpress.org. This page may be reproduced for classroom use only.

FAMILY ACTIVITY

Look at the activities in the picture below. Help your child name each activity and the body parts used for each one. Ask your child which activities he or she would like to try. Discuss how being active helps make the body strong and healthy.

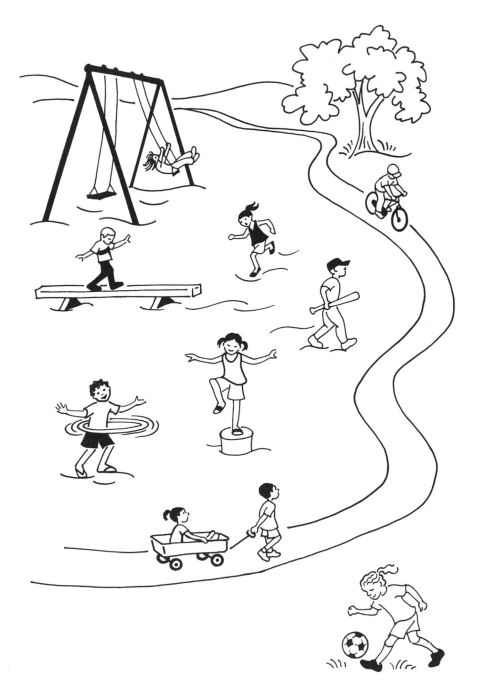

From *Fitness and Nutrition* by Connie Jo Smith, Charlotte M. Hendricks, and Becky S. Bennett, © 2014. Published by Redleaf Press, www.redleafpress.org. This page may be reproduced for classroom use only.

I Move to Be Strong!

LEARNING OBJECTIVES

- Children will communicate that physical activity helps their bodies.
- Children will participate in a variety of physical activities.
- Children will express feelings about physical activity.

Active play is essential to optimal physical development, fitness, and the overall health of young children. The benefits of active physical play throughout the day are many: increased physical development and fitness, improved weight management, increased self-esteem, and enhanced learning readiness, among many others. Young children are naturally active, learning through movement and play. Many children love to run, jump, and climb, and if encouraged, they will naturally get plenty of physical activity, building a foundation for lifelong habits. Some children, however, may need more encouragement and assistance in order to participate in movement activities.

Physical activity does not require expensive equipment or a highly structured exercise program. Large open areas provide opportunities for running, jumping, and rolling. Parachute activities promote coordination and cooperation. Walking on a wooden board placed on the ground promotes balance and coordination. Nature walks are a fun way to be physically active while integrating discovery and science activities.

The National Association for Sport and Physical Education (NASPE) has developed physical activity guidelines for young children. NASPE recommends that preschoolers participate in sixty minutes of structured physical activity and at least sixty minutes of physically active free play throughout each day. Older children should accumulate at least sixty minutes but up to several hours of age-appropriate physical activity each day. Structured activities may include games like Follow the Leader or parachute play. During free play, encourage children to alternate vigorous activities (for example, running, jumping, and rolling) and less-strenuous activities (for example, walking or exploring).

This daily accumulation of activity should include both moderate and vigorous physical activity as well as several opportunities for physical activity lasting fifteen minutes or more. Young children generally enjoy short spurts of vigorous activity, such as ten to fifteen minutes of jumping or running. These activities may be followed by quieter activities, such as sand or water play and exploring. Long, uninterrupted periods of strenuous activity (for example, adult exercise videos) are not appropriate for young children.

Aerobic activity—play that makes the heart beat faster—promotes a strong heart. Encourage children to play and move by providing opportunities to dance, move to music, play tag, jump rope, and participate in other fun physical activities. Physical play should allow for constant movement but at various activity levels—sometimes strenuous and sometimes easy.

Tracking and understanding time may be difficult for very young children. When encouraging children to engage in an activity for a specific period, identifying songs and nursery rhymes of varying lengths may be helpful. Teach these songs or rhymes, such as "The Alphabet Song," to children, and explain that they should repeat the song or rhyme a certain number of times while completing the activity. (Total time the teacher wishes the child to engage in the activity ÷ how long it takes to sing the song = number of times the song is repeated.)

Facilitate physical development, motor coordination, and fitness by supporting children when they run, jump, balance, throw balls, dance to music, and participate in other noncompetitive movement activities. Encourage all children to try a variety of activities and to develop skill and enjoyment in moving their bodies. Promote movement, activity, and fun—not competitiveness. Encourage families to participate in physical activities with their children, and remind them that physical skills and motor coordination do not improve just through aging; improvement requires demonstration, teaching, and practice.

Consider safety when encouraging movement activities. Providing a safe environment is an ongoing challenge, but it begins with age-appropriate equipment and resilient surfaces in a protected area. Wheeled toys with a wide wheelbase and a low center of gravity provide the most stability. Wading pools or areas with sprinklers should have nonslip surfaces. Swimming pool drains must have secure covers to prevent powerful and dangerous suction.

Supervision is essential to children's safety. Every child should be within sight and voice reach of a supervising adult. Be aware of children's abilities, and encourage or redirect activities to help children be successful and safe. The staff–child ratio should be consistent throughout the day, including during outdoor play; but some activities, such as water play, require additional supervision. A child can drown in a few inches of water.

Incorporate safety education daily by guiding children to take turns and to use equipment appropriately. Integrate social skills and safety while providing opportunities to promote fitness.

VOCABULARY

adventure	exercise	muscle	sweat
aerobic	fit	obstacle	train
athlete	fitness	repetition	weights
breathing	game	sport	workout
condition	gym	stopwatch	
dance	heart	strength	
endurance	jog	strong	

CREATING THE ENVIRONMENT

- Designate play spaces, both indoors and outdoors, that are large enough to accommodate all children so they have freedom of movement. Areas should be obstacle-free to prevent tripping. Inspect your play area daily, and remove debris or other potential hazards (for example, stinging insects).

- Make sure outdoor areas are enclosed with fencing or other barriers.

- Make sure playgrounds meet U.S. Consumer Product Safety Commission guidelines and criteria of the Americans with Disabilities Act. An approved resilient surface under and around equipment is as important as the equipment itself.

- Provide dense shade in outdoor play areas to extend the time of day when outside play is comfortable and to prevent overexposure to the sun's ultraviolet rays. Plan for a variety of activities when creating the environment. Tricycle paths, grassy areas for running and playing, and areas for digging each contribute to a diverse outdoor environment and promote fun physical activity.

EVALUATION

- Do children make statements about or indicate that physical activity helps their bodies?

- Do children participate in a variety of physical activities (for example, exercise, sports, and dance)?

- Are children having fun during physical activities?

- Do children show or say how they feel after physical activity (for example, feeling tired, good, or happy)?

- Do children experience physical activity throughout the day (for example, when indoors and outdoors, during free play, and when integrated with music)?

CHILDREN'S ACTIVITIES

Obstacle Course

Consider the best path for an outside obstacle course, making sure to avoid areas with heavy foot traffic and moving equipment. Build an obstacle course within the defined path using a variety of materials that are safe and age appropriate. With children's help, create signs—with pictures and words—that show which type of movement is suggested at each point along the course (for example, running, skipping, hopping, dancing, crawling, or climbing). Signs can be laminated for durability and reuse. Post each sign next to the appropriate area on the course. Before children try the course, explain that not everyone will be able to do all activities in the obstacle course, but everyone will be allowed to explore ways to use the course to increase their skills. Encourage each child to find ways to participate.

After the initial course setup and use, work with children to redesign the obstacle course on a daily or weekly basis. Encourage children to complete the course repeatedly for a certain amount of time each day, and challenge them to see if they can improve their speed of completion. Provide a stopwatch or a clock with a large face so children can capture their times. Have children record their activity completion times on a chart.

MATERIALS

- materials for building an obstacle course (for example, boxes of all sizes, climbing blocks, inner tubes, rope, rubber mats, clean tires, and old chair or sofa cushions that have been appropriately cleaned), a stopwatch or clock, paper, and pencils

❗ Safety Note: Be aware that rubber tires contain volatile organic compounds (VOCs) and may also contain heavy metals—do not use tires that are deteriorating.

OTHER IDEAS

- In a multipurpose room or other designated indoor area, create an indoor obstacle course.

- Take children to see a track meet, cross-country race, or other sporting event that incorporates movement. Have children discuss the athletes and activities they saw during the event.

- Make a video or audio recording of children explaining what movements or activities they engaged in while completing the obstacle course, how the movements made them feel, and which body parts they used.

- Provide art supplies, and ask children to sculpt or draw a person running (or jumping or climbing).

My Fitness Chart

Create a weekly chart for display that vertically lists each child's name (or photograph) along the left-hand side and horizontally lists physical activities (such as running, climbing, dancing, skipping, hopping, and jumping) along the top. If possible, create the chart on a reusable surface so you can clean it and use the chart each week. After periods of group physical activity (inside or out), ask each child to put a check mark to the right of his name (or photograph) in the column that shows the physical activity he completed during the group activity. At the end of each day or week, ask children to determine how many check marks they have for each activity and how many total check marks they have for the day or week. Provide assistance as needed.

MATERIALS

- interactive whiteboard, dry-erase board, or laminated poster board; markers; and children's photographs (if desired)

OTHER IDEAS

- Encourage children to run in place, jump up and down, or hop from foot to foot for increasing intervals. Start with fifteen seconds of activity, and then pause to rest. Repeat the activity for thirty seconds, and then pause to rest. Repeat the activity for sixty seconds. Ask children how the activity made them feel during each length of time (for example, happy, excited, tired, sleepy, and so on).

- Try the previous activity on a different day. After each interval, ask children to listen to one another's heartbeats, feel one another's pulses, and watch to see if their breathing is faster after the activity. Have children discuss their findings.

- Encourage children to create a "My Fitness Plan" (which can be a verbal or drawn plan) at the beginning of the day (or the beginning of each outside time). Ask them to indicate how many times or for how long they will jump, hop, run, and so on during outside time.

- Take a video of or photograph each of the children while they engage in a physical activity on their fitness plan. Encourage them to take their videos or photographs home to share with their families.

Dance Freeze Frame

During inside group time, play music and ask children to dance until you stop the music. Explain that when the music stops, they are to freeze in position. While in the freeze position, ask children to observe how everyone's legs and arms are positioned. Play the music for specific intervals (for example, fifteen, twenty, thirty, or sixty seconds). During some of the freeze times, take pictures of the group, noting the length of dance time prior to freezing for each picture. After the activity, discuss with the children the various body positions shown in the photos, the length of time they danced prior to each photo, how they felt during the dance, and what they liked most about the activity.

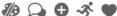

MATERIALS

- various types of music (including music from different cultures, from a variety of instruments, and of various speeds and styles), an audio device for music, and a camera

OTHER IDEAS

- Show samples of dance or music videos to the children. Divide them into small groups, and ask each group to choose music, design costumes, choreograph a dance routine, and perform their dance for the other groups.

- Watch a dance or music video with the children, and ask them to observe and count how many times people run, hop, skip, jump, or kick. Pause the video occasionally, and ask children to try to mimic certain movements they have just viewed.

- Invite a dancer or dance instructor to perform in the classroom and to teach a few moves to the children.

- Choose music of various lengths, and encourage children to dance until the song ends. Start with music that is slow and of short duration, and then use music of increasing speeds and lengths.

  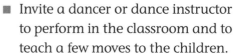

Skip, Hop, Boogie

Play a variation of musical chairs, asking children to skip, hop on one leg, jump with both feet, or dance ("boogie") around a circle of chairs until the music stops. Have children grab a seat when the music stops. Include enough seating to allow *all* children to participate. Do *not* remove seating after each round; continue to allow all children to play. Change the required movements in each round, or keep them the same.

MATERIALS

- chairs (standard child-size chairs, beanbag chairs, or individual mats), music, and an audio device for music

OTHER IDEAS

- Vary the activity by having children—after the music stops—run to a designated spot and back to the chairs before claiming one.

- Have children form pairs, and complete the activity while holding hands with a partner.

- While the music is playing, call out various movements (for example, touching toes, wiggling fingers, raising both arms, and clapping hands) for children to do when the music stops, in addition to the required movement.

  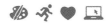

- Take the game outside and use carpet squares, cardboard pieces, or old placemats as the designated seating (or standing) spaces.

  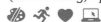

In the Zone

Create various spaces—or "zones"—where certain activities will be repeated for a certain number of times or for a certain length of time. Include zones for jumping, running, climbing, dancing, skipping, and other physical activities. In the jumping zone, have children jump from one mat or designated point to another, jump from one tire to another, jump over a series of blocks, or jump on a minitrampoline. In the running zone, ask children to run in a circle, run around objects along a marked path, or run in place. In the climbing zone, have children climb up the ladder of a sliding board, climb up or across stacked tires, or climb up a cargo net that is attached to playground equipment. The dancing zone might incorporate playing a Wii or Xbox dancing game, dancing to a variety of music, or following instructions for dance games from a book, such as *101 Dance Games for Children* by Paul Rooyackers. Activities in the skipping zone might include skipping with a rope, skipping along a designated path, or skipping to music.

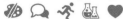

MATERIALS

- rubber mats, clean tires, large building blocks, a minitrampoline, cardboard boxes, aWii or Xbox, dancing games, an audio device for music, jump ropes, and a book of dance games

- ❗ Safety Note: Be aware that rubber tires contain volatile organic compounds (VOCs) and may also contain heavy metals—do not use tires that are deteriorating.

OTHER IDEAS

- Invite a jump rope team to the classroom to teach children basic rope jumping skills.

- Hold hopping, galloping, or skipping events on a designated course.

- Visit a gym or public playground with a variety of climbing equipment, and allow children to explore it.

- Have children measure, record, and display the distance of running paths or the distance between jump targets or activity zones.

  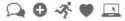

Flying High

Allow each child to carry a Styrofoam, plastic, cardboard, or paper airplane while running a specified distance away from and then back to the group. Next, give each child a piece of tape with her initials or name written on it. Then allow children to take turns flying an airplane. Each child will run to where her plane landed, mark the landing spot with her piece of tape, and then run back to the group with her plane, giving it to the next person in line. After each child has had a turn to fly a plane and mark her landing spot, help children measure and record the distances flown by the planes.

MATERIALS

- model airplanes (more than one type and style if possible), masking tape, string, measuring tape or a yardstick, paper, and markers

OTHER IDEAS

- Provide children with containers of bubbles, instructions and ingredients for making a bubble solution, or a bubble machine. Set a clock or time limit, and encourage children to chase and capture as many flying bubbles as possible. Have them count the number of bubbles they capture.

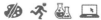

- Provide paper, decorating materials, and instructions for folding paper airplanes. Have children fold and decorate airplanes. Encourage children to flight-test their designs and to record which designs fly the farthest.

- Watch a video about how to construct a kite. Select one of many YouTube videos, such as the one at www .youtube.com/watch?v=foFeNdB2GDY.

Separate children into small groups, give kite-making and decorating materials to each group, and have each group construct a kite. Allow children in each group to take turns running with their kites.

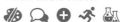

- Provide materials to small groups for constructing and decorating a superhero cape (one cape for each group). Encourage children to play tag or hide-and-seek, having the child who is "it" select one of the capes to wear while being "it."

- ❗ Safety Note: Use tape to secure capes to children's shirts. Do not allow children to run if the capes are tied around their necks.

FAMILY INFORMATION

I MOVE TO BE STRONG!

Children are naturally active and learn through movement and play. Running, jumping, crawling, and climbing help children develop strong muscles and bones. Regular physical activity helps their bodies stay healthy and fight off germs that cause sicknesses. While children are moving and having fun, they are also releasing energy and stress. Overall, children feel better when they are moving their bodies!

Children need several opportunities for physical activity each day. Young children may be able to run and jump vigorously for about fifteen minutes before they need time to relax. Later, they will be ready to run and jump again!

SAFE PLAY AREAS

Be sure your child's play area is safe. Teach your child to play away from streets and parking lots. If your child plays in a driveway or alley, always walk all around your vehicle and look for your child before starting your vehicle.

You or another adult should always watch your child when she or he is playing outdoors. It is even better if you play with your child! Here are some fun ideas:

- Walk to explore your neighborhood, or hike in the woods.

- Practice throwing, kicking, and catching a large ball.

- Dance to your favorite music.

- March around the house, or play Follow the Leader.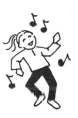

- Jump through sprinklers and water hoses on hot days.

- Run, jump, and play tag.

- Roll down a grassy hill.

From *Fitness and Nutrition* by Connie Jo Smith, Charlotte M. Hendricks, and Becky S. Bennett, © 2014.
Published by Redleaf Press, www.redleafpress.org. This page may be reproduced for classroom use only.

FAMILY ACTIVITY

Make multiple copies of this page, or put a clear wrap over the top of this page so you can reuse the table each month. Work with your child to circle two or three activities he or she might enjoy doing each week. Help your child decide how many times or how long each activity will be performed daily, and put that number in the activity box for the day. If needed, help your child keep count or keep time during the activity. Each week suggest adding another activity or increasing the amount of time or number of times the activity is performed.

Week _____ **or** **Dates:** _____

	Monday	Tuesday	Wednesday	Thursday	Friday	Saturday	Sunday

From *Fitness and Nutrition* by Connie Jo Smith, Charlotte M. Hendricks, and Becky S. Bennett, © 2014. Published by Redleaf Press, www.redleafpress.org. This page may be reproduced for classroom use only.

My Body Needs Rest!

LEARNING OBJECTIVES

- Children will express feelings about rest time and sleep time.
- Children will state reasons they need rest.
- Children will practice relaxation activities.

Most young children need to rest or relax at some time during the day. Without adult guidance to rest, children may become exhausted, overstimulated, or stressed without being aware of how they are feeling. Physical exhaustion and overstimulation increase stress, and the resulting change in a child's energy level is often misjudged by adults and treated as misbehavior. Helping children learn to recognize when they are tired or stressed and teaching them how to rest or relax may help reduce inappropriate behaviors and, in some cases, physical illnesses.

Programs may schedule a rest period, or they may encourage children to rest whenever they need to. Some children go to sleep easily, while others may only rest. Some children may be unable to rest quietly if they already have had adequate rest, if they are just too excited about other activities, or if they fear the dark or being alone. If a child cannot rest, provide time and a space for quiet play, such as looking at books or coloring.

Establish a routine when preparing for rest time. Encourage children to help with placing cots and getting their sheets or blankets from their individual storage spaces. Lowering the lights and playing soft music can create a soothing environment. Read, sing quietly, or provide other relaxation activities leading into and during rest time.

To ensure children's safety and adequate supervision, the staff–child ratio should remain constant during rest time. Check state and local licensing requirements for regulations regarding cots, sheets, length of rest periods, removal of children's shoes during rest time, cleaning and sanitation procedures, and other requirements. Position cots so that adults have visual and physical access to each child and clear exit pathways are in place.

VOCABULARY

calm	glow	relax	vibrate
cushion	inhale	rest	whistle
dark	massage	signing	wind down
dim	night-light	sleep	wind up
exhale	pillow	stretch	
exhausted	pressure	tired	
flashlight	reflection	unwind	

CREATING THE ENVIRONMENT

- Create an unrushed daily schedule that has appropriate expectations for children and a balance between active and quiet times to promote rest and relaxation.

- Designate a quiet area where a child can go to rest or play alone while remaining visible to the supervising adult. Soft, washable cushions or soft mats and a feeling of privacy make the space more inviting. Nonpoisonous plants and soft colors can provide a soothing effect.

- During rest time, dim the lighting, but do not turn it off. Quiet, soothing music may contribute to relaxation, but music from a radio station may be disruptive due to voice variations. Because water has a calming effect, water fountains, audio recordings of water sounds, and aquariums can enhance the rest time environment.

- Provide each child with a clean cot or mat for resting and a seasonally appropriate covering, such as a sheet or blanket. Space children as far away as possible from one another, or alternate children head to feet to reduce disease transmission from coughing or sneezing. Place cots in a manner that allows easy access to each child and maintains emergency exit routes.

- Be sensitive to children's needs and desires when placing cots; for example, some children may have fears that can be alleviated by placing their cots near an adult or a light source. Encourage children to bring a favorite blanket, sheet, or washable stuffed toy from home.

- Provide individual storage spaces for children's mats, blankets, and toys.

EVALUATION

- Do children role-play relaxation, rest, and sleep?

- Do children express their feelings about rest time and sleep time?

- Do children participate in routines to prepare for rest time?

- Do children participate in quiet activities during rest time if they do not sleep?

- Are children able to communicate that rest is important for their bodies?

CHILDREN'S ACTIVITIES

Wind Up and Wind Down

Show children a wind-up toy, wind it up, and then count as you watch it wind down. Ask them why they think the toy wound down or stopped. Explain to children that just as the wind-up toy wound down, our bodies get tired and run down too. Tell them that when people are tired or sleepy, they may get grouchy, rub their eyes, or yawn. Assure them that resting and sleeping help people get wound up and ready to go again. Give children wind-up toys—one for each child—and show them how to twist the keys to wind them up. Encourage them to play with the toys so they can see the process of winding up and winding down and practice counting how long it takes for the toys to wind down.

MATERIALS
- a variety of wind-up toys

OTHER IDEAS

- Help each child find a partner. Let one child pretend to be a wind-up toy while the other child pretends to wind him up. Encourage the child who is the toy to make any fast movement she chooses in the space available and then wind down to a stop. Reverse the roles.

- Show children a variety of music boxes. Wind up one of the music boxes and listen for it to wind down.

- Add a wind-up radio with a hand crank to the technology interest area for children to experience.

- Take apart a wind-up toy, and let children examine the inside working parts. Add the toy to the science and math interest area for further examination and discussion about what makes it go.

Pillow Talk

Collect a variety of pillows and cushions, and place them throughout a designated area. Encourage children to explore and learn about the pillows. Once they have had an opportunity to see and feel the pillows, ask open-ended questions like, "What do you think about the pillows?" and "How do you think pillows can be used?" Explain to children that pillows provide comfort to help people rest. Explain that people need rest to help their bodies grow strong and to help them keep moving after resting. Let them know that there are many ways, times, and places that people rest. Tell children to use the pillows to get comfortable. Play the instrumental version of "Voyage for Dreamers" by Pamala Ballingham or other soothing music while they rest. Leave out a few pillows and tell children they can use them whenever they need help to rest.

MATERIALS

- a variety of washable pillows and cushions (including many sizes, shapes, colors, textures, levels of firmness, and patterns and those with removable and permanent covers), a recording of the instrumental version of "Voyage for Dreamers" by Pamala Ballingham or some other soothing music, and an audio device for music

OTHER IDEAS

- Give each child a pillowcase and supplies to decorate it in any way he chooses.

- Engage children in making small pillows for the dolls and toy people in the dramatic play interest area. Simple no-stitch pillows can be made by decorating socks, stuffing them with scrap cloth strips, and tying the open end with ribbon. Using rulers to measure for the best size pillows and cutting socks accordingly adds a math component.

- Provide craft sticks, tree branches, scraps of cloth material, yarn, and other supplies to encourage children to construct miniature beds, hammocks, couches, and other furniture for resting.

- Read and discuss *No Nap* by Eve Bunting. Play the song "Not Naptime" by Justin Roberts, and encourage children to listen to the words. Ask children to share how they feel about naps and resting.

In and Out

Blow up a beach ball. Show children how you breathe in and then blow out air from your lungs, through your mouth, and into the beach ball to inflate it. Let them feel the air as it escapes the beach ball. Guide children to breathe in slowly through their noses and then breathe out through their mouths. Tell them to put their hands in front of their mouths to feel the air flow out. Let them know that breathing in is called *inhaling* and breathing out is called *exhaling*. Encourage them to take slow, long, and deep breaths and to exhale completely. Make a soft sighing sound while exhaling, and see if they can too. Next, invite children to stretch up as they inhale and bend down as they exhale. Briefly explain that breathing deeply and slowly can help them relax and is one way to rest and help their bodies get stronger.

MATERIALS
- a beach ball

OTHER IDEAS

- Whistle a short tune for children or play "Whistle While You Work" by Adriana Caselotti (from Walt Disney's *Snow White and the Seven Dwarfs*). Let children know that when people whistle, they are blowing air out of their mouths, similar to exhaling.

- Show children how to blow air onto a nonbreakable mirror to fog it up. Demonstrate and discuss how blowing air with your mouth open is different from blowing air with your mouth in a position to whistle.

- Provide enough wands and bubble solution for everyone to blow bubbles. Encourage children to inhale and then exhale as they blow bubbles.

- Invite a yoga instructor or practitioner to teach children a few simple poses to help them relax and breathe deeply. Encourage the instructor to show yoga tools she uses, such as mats, blocks, belts, or music.

Bodywork

Ask children if they ever rub a place on their bodies that hurts to make it feel better. Explain that massage therapists help people relax, rest, and feel better by stretching and rubbing their muscles and joints. Demonstrate using one hand to slowly massage the other hand, and instruct children to do the same with their hands. Remind them to massage every finger, their thumbs, the top of their hands, and their palms. Encourage children to rub in circles and straight lines, softly and with more pressure, and using taps to see what feels best to them. Then suggest that children use both hands to massage their own legs and feet. Let children decide whether they want to work in pairs to massage one another's feet.

MATERIALS

■ none

OTHER IDEAS

■ Introduce children to some commercial massage tools designed for home use, such as massaging sandals, vibrating pillows, footbath massagers, massage sticks, foot rollers, porcupine balls, and Jacknobbers. Have children predict how using each tool might feel, and then let them try out the tools.

■ Demonstrate how simple items can be used for massaging; for example, a rolled towel can be pulled gently back and forth around the back of the neck, a tennis ball can be rolled back and forth under the feet, a two-liter bottle can be filled with sand and rolled on legs, and playdough or clay can be squeezed with hands. Encourage everyone to try these tools.

■ Invite a massage therapist or physical therapist to explain his job and show some of the tools and techniques he uses to help people relax and strengthen their bodies.

■ Let children soak their feet in individual washtubs or bowls of warm water and two drops of lavender oil. Encourage them to talk about the smell of the lavender and the way the warm water feels on their feet.

Dancing Lights

Announce to children that you want them to make light "dance" by shining flashlights all around the ceiling, the walls, and the floor. Tell them that you are going to dim the lights and play some music while they make the light dance. Explain that they never should shine their flashlights into anyone's eyes, as that could hurt. Have each child get a throw pillow and a flashlight and find a place on the floor to rest, and then dim the overhead lights. Assist children in turning their flashlights on and off as needed. Play "Sky Dances" by Holly Near, and encourage children to be creative with their flashlight dancing. After the song ends, turn up the overhead lights to full brightness, and have children return their pillows and flashlights to the designated spaces. Ask them what they thought of the dancing lights.

MATERIALS

- throw pillows, flashlights, a recording of "Sky Dances" by Holly Near, and an audio device for music

OTHER IDEAS

- Place transparent colored film, tissue paper, or paper doilies over the flashlights, attaching the material to the flashlights with rubber bands. Have children explore how these materials affect the light as they shine it into dark spaces.

- Attend a light show, fireworks display, or performance theater to see the lighting.

- Show children a variety of night-lights, and explore how they work. Initiate a discussion about how some people are afraid of the dark and how night-lights may help. Plug in the night-lights throughout the room while children are away. When they return, let children know that you are going to dim the lights. Go on a slow and safe search for night-lights. Play the song "Night Light" by Justin Roberts, and listen to the words.

    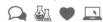

- Add a variety of flashlights and batteries to the science and math interest area, and encourage children to place batteries into flashlights and test them.

❶ Safety Note: Use flashlights with large batteries rather than button-size batteries, which could be swallowed and are choking and toxicity hazards. Ensure that batteries are new and in good shape with no rust or acid leaks that could be hazardous.

Glow Show

Ask children if they have seen anything glow in the dark, and listen to their experiences. Tell them you have some art supplies to help them make glow-in-the-dark posters. Ask them to talk about what they want to put on their glow-in-the-dark posters. Support children as they produce their posters. After all posters are finished and dry, plan a special "Glow Show." Let children work on invitations that will glow in the dark, and send the invitations to another class or to children's families. Also invite local media to the event. Until showtime, let children display their posters where they can see them when they rest. Let children practice showing their pictures to one another in the dark, and help any children who are afraid of the dark handle their fears. At the show, have children hold or display their posters so that all guests can see them. Ask visitors to remain seated, and dim the lights for a one-minute glow-in-the-dark poster viewing. Turn the lights back to full brightness, and invite guests to walk around and ask the artists questions about their creations. Following the show, let children take their posters home to look at when they rest there.

MATERIALS

- glow-in-the-dark art supplies or objects (such as crayons, paint, chalk, tape, stars, and stickers), poster board, glue, and other desired supplies

OTHER IDEAS

- Provide glow-in-the-dark body makeup pencils or paint and assist children in decorating their arms, legs, or faces. Let them see how they look, and encourage them to discuss their body artwork. Take photographs of them in the light and in the dark so they can compare them.

- Add glow-in-the-dark accessories, such as necklaces, bracelets, and clocks, to the dramatic play interest area.

- Show children reflective and glow-in-the-dark safety items, such as light sticks, exit signs, vests, collars and harnesses for pets, bike ankle bands, armbands for runners, road safety triangles, traffic cones with reflective collars, hard hats, reflective tape, and step thread. If items are not available, show photographs of them. Discuss the items, and explain that many activities besides sleep and rest take place in the dark.

- Read and discuss *What Was I Scared Of?*, a Glow-in-the-Dark Encounter by Dr. Seuss.

FAMILY INFORMATION

MY BODY NEEDS REST!

Children need more sleep than adults. Most young children need ten to twelve hours of sleep each night and a short nap during the day. Children need a schedule that allows them to get enough sleep. For example, if you must wake your child at seven o'clock each morning, then bedtime should be by eight-thirty each evening. Stay on schedule as much as possible, even on weekends.

Some children resist bedtime and sleep. Often the more tired they are, the more they try to stay awake. Children will fall asleep more quickly if they have a routine that allows them to relax before bedtime. This routine may include taking a bath, brushing teeth, reading a story, getting a last drink of water, and lots of hugs.

Lower the Lights

Many children are afraid of the dark, of noises, and of thunderstorms. These fears are very real to children. A night-light or lamp can help some children feel more secure. Playing soft music may help a child who is afraid of "monsters," as may closing closet doors and checking under the bed.

Assure your child that you will be home while he or she sleeps. Leave your child's bedroom door open so your child knows you can hear her or him if needed. Allow your child to sleep with a favorite washable toy or blanket.

Bad Dreams

Some children have difficulty sleeping because of bad dreams or night terrors. These dreams may be caused by seeing or experiencing a frightening event. Watching scary television shows or hearing adults talk about violent or dangerous events can scare children. Even children's stories and fairy tales can frighten some children.

Nightmares are very real to a child. If you know what frightens your child, you can probably prevent some bad dreams in the future.

From *Fitness and Nutrition* by Connie Jo Smith, Charlotte M. Hendricks, and Becky S. Bennett, © 2014. Published by Redleaf Press, www.redleafpress.org. This page may be reproduced for classroom use only.

FAMILY ACTIVITY

Cut out the items at the bottom of the page. Allow your child to color the large picture below. Once your child has finished coloring, talk to him or her about bedtime and rest time and how we all need rest to have energy and feel good. Discuss items your child likes to have when lying down to rest, and then let your child place the cut-out pictures on the large picture to help the child in the image rest too!

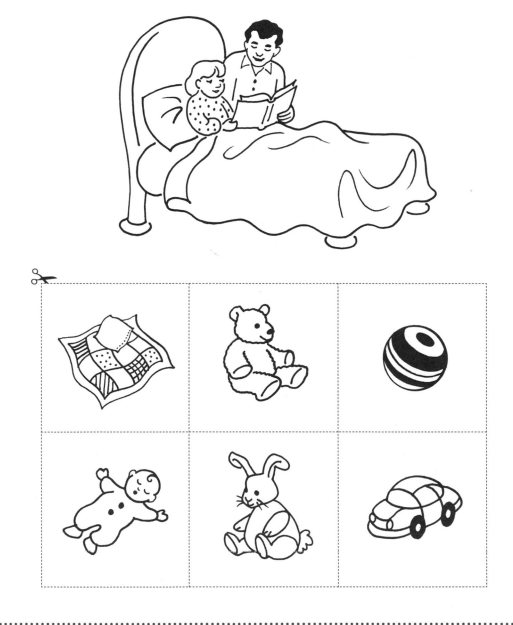

From *Fitness and Nutrition* by Connie Jo Smith, Charlotte M. Hendricks, and Becky S. Bennett, © 2014.
Published by Redleaf Press, www.redleafpress.org. This page may be reproduced for classroom use only.

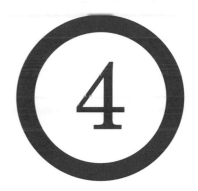

Sometimes I Rumble and Roar!

LEARNING OBJECTIVES

- Children will describe ways they know they are hungry or thirsty (for example, feeling their stomachs growl, feeling empty, and having a dry mouth).

- Children will indicate signs of fullness.

- Children will communicate that their bodies need food and water.

Lifelong eating habits are shaped during children's early years, so teachers have a special opportunity to lay the foundation for sound eating habits and to help children establish a healthy relationship with food. Providing nutritionally balanced meals and snacks and integrating nutrition education and healthful eating habits in the home and early childhood environment can help prevent health risks such as childhood obesity.

When infants are hungry, they cry. Being fed and having their hunger alleviated are usually the results of their crying. Further, infants learn they not only receive food and feel better when they cry, but they also receive comfort and security as they are held and cuddled. As children grow, they can learn to recognize specific needs, such as being hungry and needing food. They can also recognize feelings, such as being sad and needing a hug. To help children make the connection between hunger and food, promote the idea that food is for hunger rather than reward or comfort.

Help children become aware of and responsible for their bodies by teaching them skills such as hand washing and toothbrushing. Use the same approach for teaching self-regulation of eating as you do for teaching hygiene practices—that is, teach children to listen to their bodies' signs, in this case signs of hunger and fullness. As children learn their own body cues for hunger and fullness, encourage them to communicate when they are full and hungry and to demonstrate their understanding through mealtime serving and eating practices. Adults are responsible for providing nutritious, appetizing food in an appropriate setting; children can decide how much or even whether they eat.

Children generally eat only what pleases them on a specific day. Some children may eat only one or two food items, and some children may eat a lot on one day and a little the next. For most toddlers and preschool children, hunger occurs about every two and a half to three hours. Young children have small stomachs that cannot hold as much food as an adult's can. Offer nutritious, appetizing choices of food, and help children self-serve appropriate portions of each food. Help children begin to understand portion control, and encourage them to take appropriate portions. Some children may want to take large amounts of favorite foods. They may be more comfortable taking small portions if they know they can have second servings when they still feel hungry. Serve all foods at one time, and allow children to eat foods in the order they prefer.

Children must have water available to them throughout the day, including during outside playtime and on field trips. Children lose fluid from their bodies throughout the day but especially when participating in vigorous play (such as running and jumping) and during warm weather. They can become dehydrated very quickly, leading to a potentially dangerous health condition.

As children learn their hunger cues, they also begin to recognize when they are thirsty. Thirst is an important concept; many people (including adults) mistake thirst for hunger, resulting in unnecessary overeating. Water is the best thirst quencher; avoid sweetened beverages and carbonated soda (which contains acid), energy drinks, and caffeinated beverages. While 100 percent juice contains valuable nutrients, it also contains calories and acid; limit the amount of juice children consume daily, and serve juice with meals or snacks. Water also may be available at mealtimes, but water should not replace milk as required by nutrition guidelines.

Young children cannot begin to understand the digestive process, but they can begin to understand that their bodies need food and water. Many children find it fascinating to be introduced to what happens to food and water after they are swallowed.

VOCABULARY

chew	empty	hungry	parched
dehydrated	famished	ice	portion
digestion	full	liquid	ravenous
drink	gas	meal	serving
eat	growl	nutritious	snack

solid	swallow	water
starving	thirsty	

CREATING THE ENVIRONMENT

- Provide children with a variety of nutritious, appetizing food choices. Meals that allow children to select the food and serve themselves may encourage them to try new foods and take responsibility for their food choices. Provide assistance, as necessary, to help children choose appropriate-size portions.

- Provide child-size tables and chairs so young children can easily reach the table while sitting comfortably with their feet touching the floor. Small trays, plates, and cups make grasping, lifting, and carrying easier for children.

- Encourage a homelike environment by involving children in passing serving bowls and serving themselves. Occasionally use place mats, tablecloths, centerpieces, and cloth napkins to make the table setting attractive and to show children a variety of table settings.

- Have cool water available to children throughout the day. Water fountains should be child-size. If child-size fountains are not possible, provide sturdy nonslip stepstools for children to use.

EVALUATION

- Do children talk about what being hungry and thirsty feel like?
- Do children slow down or stop eating when they are full?
- Are words such as *hungry, thirsty,* and *full* used during play?
- Do children talk about how their bodies use food?
- Do children request or get a drink of water when they are thirsty?

CHILDREN'S ACTIVITIES

What Does *Hungry* Mean?

Select any doll or toy person, and introduce her to children as Rosita. Tell them she is hungry. Ask children what they think *hungry* means and what Rosita should do. Listen to their ideas and suggestions. Show a hardback or online children's dictionary, and read what it says under *hungry*. Encourage children to share stories about being hungry. Explain that everyone gets hungry sometimes and that eating when hungry is important. End the activity by letting children know where you are going to put Rosita so they can feed her and her friends (other dolls or toy people) whenever they are hungry.

MATERIALS

- any doll or toy person, a children's hardback or online dictionary (for example, www.wordsmyth.net or www.factmonster.com), additional dolls and toy people (include both male and female dolls that represent different ethnic backgrounds)

OTHER IDEAS

- Encourage children to dictate or write poems or stories about being hungry. Encourage children to illustrate their creations. Providing a first line for the poem may help children begin.

- Have children act out being hungry.

- Arrange for children to interview a veterinarian or pet owner to find out how animals show hunger. Help children come up with questions in advance.

- Read and discuss *The Very Hungry Caterpillar* by Eric Carle.

The Lion's Roar

Show children a toy lion or a photograph of a lion, and play the sound of a lion roaring. Alternately, show a video of a lion roaring. Ask children what else roars or growls. Help them think of other animals, such as dogs, tigers, and bears. Ask children to move and make the sound of any animal that roars or growls. Then ask if they have ever heard their stomachs roar or growl. Point out that they may be hungry when their stomachs growl. Tell children that sometimes the stomach muscles start to move at the times they usually eat, even if they haven't eaten yet. Explain that the movement sounds like a growl or rumble. Encourage them to listen to their stomachs and other people's stomachs for growls.

MATERIALS

- a toy lion or a photograph of a lion, a recording of a roar sound from a DVD about lions or online source (such as www.sandiegozoo.org/animalbytes/t-lion.html) or a video clip of lion roaring, and an audio device or computer for playing the recording or video clip

OTHER IDEAS

- Help each child make a stethoscope by attaching funnels to each end of a plastic tube. Encourage children to listen to their own stomachs for growls or other indications that they may be hungry. Ask them to describe what they hear.

  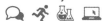

- Use real, play, or homemade stethoscopes to let children listen to one another's stomachs. Ask them to describe any sounds they hear that may indicate hunger. Tell children they need permission from a person before listening to that person's stomach.

- Read and role-play *Dinosaur Roar!* by Paul and Henrietta Stickland.

- Play and sing the song "Roar Like a Lion" by Patty Shukla, available on YouTube at www.youtube.com/watch?v=MMTTqUmC_AI.

Full to the Top

Provide children with clean sand, a variety of containers, sand scoops, and shovels. Invite them to put different amounts of sand into various containers. Have them fill some containers so full that they cannot be moved without spilling sand. Talk with the children about what *full* means. Then ask them to explain how they feel after they have eaten. Ask if they know what it feels like to eat too much. Explain that eating until they feel full is important, but they should not feel so full that they get a stomachache. As follow-up, talk with the children about the concept of full after the next time they eat.

MATERIALS

■ sand, a variety of containers (such as plastic cups, bottles, pitchers, buckets, and bowls), sand scoops, and shovels

OTHER IDEAS

■ Provide clean water and various containers for children to experiment with as they learn the concepts of empty and full. Remind children to wash their hands before and after water play.

■ Show children a clear plastic container with a large opening and more than enough same-size rocks (or Ping-Pong balls) to fill it. Ask children to guess how many rocks it will take to fill the container, and have them count together as they help you fill the container.

■ Provide several containers, such as boxes, cans, bags, and purses, with some of them full. Invite children to sort the containers into groups based on whether they are full or not full.

■ Read and discuss *The Gas We Pass: The Story of Farts* by Shinta Cho. Point out that when people eat, they also swallow air. Explain that air can make people feel full until they release it by passing gas as a burp or flatus. Show them a picture of the path of air and food.

Where Does Food Go?

Ask children where they think food goes and what they think happens to it after they eat. Listen to their ideas and write them down for all to see. After children wash their hands, give them each a banana to peel and gently feel. Ask what their teeth do to food when they eat. Give children plastic knives, and ask them to examine the knives' teeth. Then have them use the knives (on individual plates) to cut the bananas into small pieces as their teeth would.

Involve children in moving one cup of cut-up bananas into a blender or food processor. Prepare them for the loud noise, and then turn on the blender for five seconds. Stop the blender, and ask children to look at and compare the blended bananas to those not yet blended. Add a cup of milk or vanilla yogurt and two ice cubes to the blender, and blend for about thirty more seconds. After the smoothie is ready, ask children what happened to the bananas. Pour the smoothie into small cups so they can see that the bananas are no longer solid. Encourage children to taste the results. Allow children to help you use the remaining bananas to mix up smoothies for a snack. Tell children that when they chew their food, it mixes with saliva. After swallowing, the food goes to the stomach, where muscles begin to mash it up (just like the blender mashed up the bananas). Explain that the food is then sent out to feed the rest of the body. Tell them the body uses what it needs and then gets rid of the food that is not used when they go to the bathroom. Show children computer simulations, pictures, or short videos of the digestive system. As follow-up, invite children in small groups to look up digestion in resource books and on the computer with you.

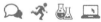

MATERIALS

- bananas, a blender or food processor, plastic or table knives, plates or cutting boards for cutting bananas, milk or vanilla yogurt, ice cubes, drinking cups, a measuring cup, digestion resource books or videos, a medical or encyclopedia website with digestion videos, and a viewing device for the videos (such as a computer)

OTHER IDEAS

- Provide clean water and clear tubes of various lengths so children can explore the movement of water as it runs from one end to the other. Remind children to wash their hands before and after playing in the water.

- Invite a medical professional to visit the classroom to show a model of the digestive system.

- Visit a sanitary landfill (or dump) or other similar location with children, and watch the trash compactor.

Explain how the trash compactor acts like our bodies when we process the food we eat.

- Read and discuss *Everyone Poops* by Taro Gomi.

Give the Plants a Drink

Select safe plants for an environment with children, and bring them to the classroom. Teach children how to observe the plants and gently touch the soil each day to check for dryness. Provide a chart for each plant so children can record the soil conditions (moist or dry). Help children measure water in a measuring cup and give the plants a drink when needed. Explain to children that all people need to drink water, just as plants do. Tell them that water helps their bodies work the right way.

❗ Safety Note: For assistance in determining which plants are safe for children's environments, consult your local poison center or call the American Association of Poison Control Centers at 1-800-222-1222.

MATERIALS
- safe plants (such as zebra plants, purple passion plants, and coleus plants), a chart to track soil conditions and watering, and a measuring cup or watering can

OTHER IDEAS
- Provide water and sand or soil for children to mix together to explore various stages of dry and moist.

- Show children a variety of containers used by animals (such as dogs, hamsters, birds, and so on) and people for drinking water. Encourage children to examine the containers to see how they work and to talk about how they are alike and different.

- Help each child make a simple rain gauge using a can or plastic jar with a large opening. Show children how to use a ruler and permanent marker to indicate the inch, half-inch, and quarter-inch marks, and then place the gauges outside where they can catch the falling rain.

- Read and discuss *Water* by Frank Asch or another book about water.

Tell Rosita

Reintroduce children to the doll (or toy person) named Rosita and some of her friends (other dolls and toy people). Tell children that Rosita and her friends have some questions about food. One at a time, pick up prepared cards that you have placed near the hands of each doll and toy person. Read the question from the card, and listen to children's answers to determine what they know about food and hunger. Use the questions in the materials list and write your own questions based on your knowledge of the children.

MATERIALS

■ dolls and toy people (including both male and female dolls that represent different ethnic backgrounds), and cards prepared with questions on them:

What does *hungry* mean?

What does *full* mean?

How do you know if you are hungry?

Why do people eat?

What does *thirsty* mean?

What should you do if you are hungry or thirsty?

What happens to food when we swallow it?

When should we stop eating?

How do you know if you are full?

OTHER IDEAS

■ Encourage children to write, illustrate, and bind (with tape or yarn or with metal rings through punched holes) a book about being hungry and thirsty.

■ Let children write and record a song about being hungry and thirsty. With children's agreement, share the audio or video recording with the group and their families. If the video is posted online in a public format (such as on YouTube or another similar site), be sure to have media releases for the children on file.

- Paste a picture of the digestive system onto cardboard, and then cut the cardboard into jigsaw pieces for children to piece together again and again.

- Give children water to drink with straws, out of cups, from bottles, and with ice. Ask them which way they like to drink water best and why.

FAMILY INFORMATION

SOMETIMES I RUMBLE AND ROAR!

Children need breakfast to get through the busy morning. After all, it has been ten or twelve hours since they last ate. Skipping breakfast can mean growling stomachs and grumpy children, and it can make doing well in school difficult.

Most young children need to eat about every two and a half to three hours. Give your child small, nutritious snacks between meals, such as fruit or peanut butter and crackers. It is okay to occasionally give your child sweets, like cookies or cake, if your child has eaten healthful foods during meals.

Young children need small servings of food (about one-fourth cup per serving). If children are served large portions of food and forced to clean their plates, they may become overweight or learn to dislike some foods.

HUNGER AND FULLNESS

Learning the signs of hunger and fullness is an important lesson for children. Adults are responsible for serving nutritious and appetizing food. Children are responsible for deciding how much they eat.

Teach your child to take small servings of foods. If he or she is still hungry, allow a second serving of some foods. Do not insist that your child eat everything on his or her plate.

DRINK WATER

Children lose fluid from their bodies when they play, especially in warm weather. Have water available for your child all day. Water is the best fluid for your child's body.

From *Fitness and Nutrition* by Connie Jo Smith, Charlotte M. Hendricks, and Becky S. Bennett, © 2014. Published by Redleaf Press, www.redleafpress.org. This page may be reproduced for classroom use only.

FAMILY ACTIVITY

Help your child choose the pictures that he or she thinks shows each of the following: hungry, full, thirsty, and empty. Ask questions such as "Why do you think
this picture shows being hungry?" and "What does hungry feel like?" Use these
descriptive words when asking questions about food and drinks. Talk with your
child about trying to recognize when she or he is hungry, thirsty, and full, and
about eating, drinking, or stopping when his or her body says it's time.

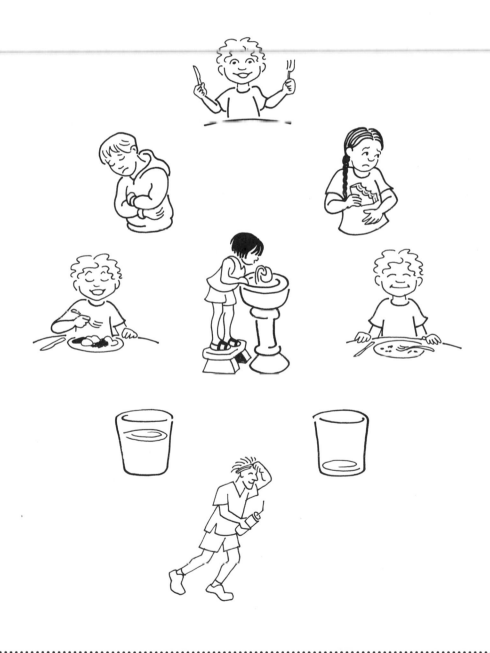

From *Fitness and Nutrition* by Connie Jo Smith, Charlotte M. Hendricks, and Becky S. Bennett, © 2014.
Published by Redleaf Press, www.redleafpress.org. This page may be reproduced for classroom use only.

My Body Needs Food to Grow and Go!

LEARNING OBJECTIVES

- Children will sort foods into different food groups (for example, by color, texture, and "anytime" foods versus "sometimes" foods).
- Children will identify foods that give our bodies what they need to grow and develop.
- Children will show respect for different eating habits (for example, those associated with family and cultural/religious patterns, food allergies, and medical requirements).

Children need basic nutrients—protein, carbohydrates, and fats—as well as vitamins and minerals to grow strong and healthy. By eating a variety of foods, most children will get the nutrition they need. It is okay if a child eats a tuna or banana sandwich every day for lunch, but offer a variety of fruits, vegetables, and other foods along with that sandwich daily.

Milk, cheese, eggs, peanut butter or sunflower-seed butter, yogurt, and lean meats are good sources of protein. Bread, oatmeal, grits, rice, cereal, and pancakes provide carbohydrates. Fruits and vegetables are loaded with vitamins and minerals. Choose fruits and vegetables in a variety of colors: yellow, green, red, white, purple, orange, and more! All foods contain some nutrients, but some foods are more healthful than others. For example, a potato provides carbohydrates, fiber, and vitamin C, plus small amounts of other nutrients. Potato chips, however, may also be loaded with more sugar, salt, and fat than the body needs. Most children do not eat large amounts of food, so provide foods that are nutritious.

Young children may not fully understand how to categorize foods into specific food groups, such as fruits, vegetables, grains, and dairy. Instead, children may enjoy sorting foods by characteristics such as color, texture, and preparation method. Encourage children to taste and enjoy a variety of foods. Think week by week, rather than day by day. Even so-called picky eaters will generally get necessary nutrients if a variety of foods are prepared and offered in appetizing and appealing ways for snacks and meals.

Encourage but do not force children to try a variety of foods. The way foods are prepared and served affects the way children feel about certain foods. Foods that are familiar, that look and smell good, and that are served in child-size portions are generally more appetizing. Children may dislike a food at one time but decide several weeks later that they like the food, or vice versa. Try to get a new food on children's tongues at least eighteen times, even if each is just a tiny taste. Try preparing and offering foods in various and creative ways. A child who does not like cooked apples may enjoy a bright red apple when sliced to reveal the "star" during a food activity. Likewise, many children are hesitant to try asparagus if it is overcooked and soft; asparagus is one of many vegetables that can be served raw with plain or flavored yogurt, light dressing, or other dips.

Children have more taste buds than adults and are therefore more sensitive to flavors. Foods with pepper or other spices may taste too hot or spicy for young children. Their food likes and dislikes may change as they grow older and the number of taste buds they have decreases.

As toddlers and preschoolers are exposed to new foods, they may begin to recognize and identify specific foods, first by color and later by food type. For example, broccoli and green beans may be categorized first as "green foods" and later as "vegetables." As children begin to understand the concepts of food identification and categorizing, you can begin to discuss how specific foods help our bodies. It is essential for children—and adults—to recognize that different foods help our bodies in different ways. Encourage children to eat a variety of foods to obtain adequate nutrients for growth and development. Whereas adults may use terms such as *nutrients*, children may better understand the concept of nutrition through description: foods can help them grow, give them energy to run and play, and help them become strong.

Some children may have special dietary needs and require different food preparation or feeding methods or a different frequency of meals. Other children may have food allergies. Allergies can cause reactions including moodiness, stomach distress, and hives—and some food reactions may be life threatening. A child who is severely allergic to peanuts, for example, may go into anaphylactic shock if exposed to peanuts, peanut butter, snack cakes or cookies containing peanuts or peanut oil, or vegetables stir-fried in peanut oil. Find out what type of reaction a child with food allergies may have and the specific food or ingredient that causes the reaction.

If a child has a potentially serious reaction to a specific food, such as peanuts, eliminating that food from the classroom environment may be necessary.

Work with the families of all children to help them understand the importance of eliminating that food in the classroom. Offer alternative foods, and provide nutrition activities that every child can enjoy.

Become familiar with the families of children in your care and in the community. Food choices, preparation methods, and eating habits are often influenced by culture and religious beliefs. Encourage and model respect for food choices.

VOCABULARY

apron	grain	oven	sweets
banquet	grill	picnic	taste
chef	kitchen	pot holder	toaster
farm	measure	recipe	vegetable
feast	meat	restaurant	
fruit	menu	slow cooker	
garden	orchard	sprout	

CREATING THE ENVIRONMENT

- Create a space for classroom cooking activities; cooking activities provide excellent opportunities to introduce new foods to children. Follow sound safety and sanitation practices when using appliances and preparing food. Set up sturdy, clean surfaces for food preparation, and find adequate storage spaces for appliances not in use. A supply of aprons, pot holders, stirring spoons, measuring spoons and cups, and utensils allows children to be directly involved in preparations.

- Serve meals and snacks family-style, helping children learn to serve themselves and encouraging them to try new foods. Create a pleasant and appealing environment during mealtimes, with conversations centered on children's interests.

- Read books and show photographs that reflect the various food choices and practices of children and families in the program and in the larger community. Add related models and props to the dramatic play interest area.

- Post information about known food allergies as reminders for staff members and volunteers. Do not include children's names or other identifying information on the posting; maintain confidentiality at all times.

EVALUATION

- Do children sort or name foods during play or while eating?
- Do children talk about foods that help their bodies?
- Do children show an interest in, taste, or eat a variety of foods when offered?

- Do children discuss what their families eat at home or foods they do not eat (for example, because of food allergies, religious beliefs, cultural patterns, or medical requirements)?

- Do children talk about their food choices or favorite foods?

CHILDREN'S ACTIVITIES

A Bundle of Bread

Ask children to recall and talk about any bread-baking or eating experiences they have had. Provide a tray of various breads that children can sample after they wash their hands. Show children the container for each kind of bread as well as the label. Read *Bread, Bread, Bread* by Ann Morris, and talk about it with the children. Let children talk about the kinds of bread they eat at home or in restaurants. Point out that many kinds of bread exist and that bread is only one kind of food. Ask children what food they eat other than bread. Write each child's name on a page in a book of blank pages bound with tape, yarn, or metal rings through punched holes. Write the foods each child names on her page. As children think of other foods, they can add them to their page in the book. Make the class book, titled *Many Kinds of Food,* available to children so they can illustrate their own pages. Place *Bread, Bread, Bread* in the library interest area or dramatic play interest area.

MATERIALS

- a tray to display bread; a wide variety of bread (including tortillas, pita bread, bagels, corn bread, rye bread, lefse, focaccia, and others); bread containers with labels; a copy of *Bread, Bread, Bread* by Ann Morris; paper; marker; tape, yarn or metal rings; and art supplies

OTHER IDEAS

- Visit a wheat, barley, corn, or oat field to learn how grains are grown and harvested and to see the machines used to prepare the earth (such as a tractor and plow), plant the seeds (such as a corn drill), and harvest the crop (such as a combine).

- Visit a grain mill, or demonstrate how a small grain mill works using a home wheat grinder, preferably one with a hand crank so children can assist. As a substitute, use a coffee grinder to show the process of grinding.

- Use a simple biscuit recipe (two cups of flour, a half cup of milk, one-fourth cup of shortening, and one tablespoon of baking powder), and let children make biscuits after they wash their hands. Allow time to gently knead and fold the dough and to shape individual biscuits, either free-form or using cookie cutters.

■ Invite a basket weaver to demonstrate basket making and to explain briefly how baskets can be used to hold food and how they are important in various cultures. In advance ask the visitor if children can handle the materials (such as the reed or cane) and tools. Add bread or fruit baskets to the dramatic play interest area and basket-making books to the language arts interest area.

Restaurant Visits

Arrange to take children to a restaurant to learn about the wide range of foods on the menu. Tell children about the restaurant they will visit and show photographs, advertisements, place mats, or coupons from the restaurant. Show a map with the restaurant marked and the roads to get there highlighted. Help children decide on questions to ask and things to observe. During the visit, encourage children to look at the menu and hear it read aloud, to notice table decorations and dishware, and to ask questions of staff members. Children may be able to take a tour of the kitchen, see equipment used to prepare food, and assist workers with simple tasks, including observing or greeting customers. Request a menu and any other restaurant materials to enhance follow-up discussions and role playing. An order of takeout food can be brought back to the program for a tasting experience. Use a camera to capture the experience, and encourage ongoing discussions and restaurant-focused dramatic play. To extend the experience, assist children in creating a restaurant in the dramatic play interest area.

MATERIALS
- menus from a restaurant; photographs, advertisements, place mats, and coupons from the restaurant; a map showing the restaurant; and a camera

OTHER IDEAS

- Visit a hotel or conference center to see the banquet halls, service stations, and kitchens. Look for artistic displays of food. Talk with children about the size of the rooms where food for large events is served.

- Show short video clips of ethnic restaurants and the food they serve. Point out the differences and similarities in the menus.

- Show sample restaurant menus and photographs of menus and sandwich boards. Provide supplies for children to create menus, menu boards, and sandwich boards.

- Set up a restaurant area for dramatic play, and add a variety of props, including pretend food, a cash register, food-order pads, tablecloths, menus, and so on.

Who Is the Cook?

Put on an apron and chef hat. If children have visited restaurants, ask them if they have seen any of the cooks. Tell them that cooks work in restaurants, but people also cook at home. Ask children who cooks where they live. On a board or chart paper, write each child's name, and draw stick people to represent the number of people each child reports as a cook. Engage all children in counting the number of stick people per child, and then add an equal sign and the appropriate numeral next to the stick people. Count the stick people for the total group, and add an equal sign and the appropriate numeral. Ask children what foods are cooked where they live. Consider presenting a variety of food photographs for children to select from when identifying foods they eat with their families. Reinforce acceptance of the various people who cook in each family and the various foods cooked. Help children see the differences and similarities of the foods eaten by their families. Encourage children to draw a picture of the cooks in their families. Display the drawings on a bulletin board. Offer to write the names of the cooks and the foods on children's drawings.

MATERIALS
- an apron, a chef hat, a board or chart paper, a marker, and art supplies (including skin-tone crayons, a range of skin-tone construction paper, and manila drawing paper)

OTHER IDEAS
- Set up a display of grills, rice cookers, toaster ovens, toasters, slow cookers, and other small appliances used for preparing food. Encourage children to compare these items. Explain that cooks may use some of the appliances but may also have specialty equipment.

- Visit the host of a local cooking show or segment on a local news channel. Arrange for a backstage pass so children can learn about the tools used to produce the show as well as the job of the cook.

- Invite family members to visit and demonstrate cooking a dish, or invite them to bring a favorite food for children to sample. Obtain information about ingredients in the dish beforehand to ensure substitutions can be incorporated for children with allergies or cultural beliefs that would prohibit them from sampling the shared food.

■ Invite cooks from the program, local professional chefs from restaurants, or instructors from a cooking school to visit the classroom, talk about their jobs, and show tools used in their work. Ask the cooks to talk about the kinds of food they prepare.

Limas, Pintos, and Garbanzos

Explain to children that beans are a type of food that helps their bodies grow strong. Provide children with uncooked mixed dried beans to sort. Tell them that even though the beans look different from one another, they are all still beans. Encourage children to sort the beans by color, size, shape, texture, weight, known varieties, and unknown varieties. Invite children to use the beans to outline the letters in their names, to order the beans from largest to smallest, to count the beans, and to create designs with the beans. Provide photographs of cooked beans from recipes, cans, or bags for children to see and use in play. Involve children in washing and preparing the beans for cooking, and then serve the beans for lunch.

❗ Safety Note: Red kidney beans, lima beans, and some other types of beans are poisonous before they are cooked. Select beans carefully. Supervise carefully children who may put small objects, like beans, into their mouths, noses, or ears.

MATERIALS
■ uncooked mixed dried beans (including northern, pinto, large lima, black-eyed, garbanzo, small white, baby lima, white kidney, cranberry bean, pink bean, black bean, navy, soybean, and adzuki), clean and empty food containers with photographs of cooked beans, and photographs of cooked beans on recipes

OTHER IDEAS
■ Help children sprout dried beans using bean seeds, moist paper towels, clean plastic bags or cups, and sunshine. Monitor and record the growth on a chart. Check with local cooperative extension system offices for current safety information and guidance.

■ Provide small containers and soil for children to plant bean seeds. Monitor and record the growth on a chart.

■ Have a bean-tasting party that includes a wide range of cooked bean dishes. For each dish prepared, provide an index card with the name of the dish, the type of bean included, and a few glued-on dried beans.

■ Read and act out *Growing Vegetable Soup* by Lois Ehlert.

Planning a Picnic

Ask children to tell you what they know about picnics, and involve them in planning one. Together, list all the things that need to be done to get ready for the picnic. The list might include choosing a location, arranging transportation, scheduling, checking weather reports, designing a backup plan in the case of bad weather, making invitations for families and friends, identifying the number of participants and the quantity of food needed, selecting a menu, preparing food, figuring out sanitation and hand-washing procedures, planning recreation, selecting music, and preparing for cleanup. Small groups of children can work on various jobs and share their progress with the group periodically. Support small groups, and facilitate the picnic planning as needed.

MATERIALS

- a computer or art materials to create invitations, a calendar, the weather report, baskets and food containers, premoistened wipes and hand sanitizer, picnic food, drinks, a cooler with ice, games, and trash bags

OTHER IDEAS

- Invite family members to visit the classroom to share some of their family traditions related to food. Ask each visitor if picnicking is something his family does together.

- Into an open picnic basket, place a wide range of photographs of food and food containers with labels. Cover the basket with a cloth napkin. Let each child put her hand under the napkin and remove one photo or container without looking. Ask the child to talk about the food on the container or in the photo.

- With children, plan a picnic for the classroom dolls and toy people. Count the dolls and toy people, and conduct an inventory of the pretend food available to determine if more is needed.

- Read and discuss books about picnics, such as *The Teddy Bears' Picnic* by Jimmy Kennedy.

Group the Food

Ask children to find photographs of food in catalogs and magazines. Have them cut out the photographs and glue each picture to a separate paper plate. Once children have created a large collection of food on paper plates, encourage them to sort the pictures in many ways; for example, children can sort according to color, size, texture, known and unknown foods, and likes and dislikes, or they can sort based on whether the food is chewy or crunchy, a food or a drink, a vegetable or a fruit, a dessert or a main course, hot or cold, cooked or raw, soft or hard, and so on. Add these plates to the dramatic play interest area for use in role playing.

MATERIALS

- magazines and catalogs with photographs of food, paper plates, and glue or paste

OTHER IDEAS

- Visit a vegetable garden, orchard, or farm to see how food is grown and to learn about the equipment used in the process. Ask in advance if children can help with watering, weeding, picking, or another task.

- Visit the produce section of a grocery store, farmers' market, or natural foods store to see the wide variety of food. Point out how the food is displayed and the tools used to keep the food fresh.

- Invite a potter to visit the classroom to show pieces that could be used to hold food. Talk about the kinds of food that would be appropriate for each dish (such as for a bowl, a plate, a cup, a pitcher, and so on). If possible, let children see the tools used to make pottery. Encourage children to use clay in the art interest area to replicate the pottery they saw.

- Throughout the indoor environment, add artwork focusing on food. Consider replicas of the work of famous artists, such as *Still Life with Apples* by Paul Cézanne, *The Pink Tablecloth* by Henri Matisse, *Wheatfield with Crows* by Vincent van Gogh, and *Campbell's Soup Cans* by Andy Warhol.

FAMILY INFORMATION

MY BODY NEEDS FOOD TO GROW AND GO!

Children need basic nutrients—protein, carbohydrates, and fats—as well as vitamins and minerals to grow strong and healthy. By eating a variety of foods, most children will get what they need. It is okay if your child wants a serving of macaroni and cheese every day; just make sure he or she also eats fruits, vegetables, and other dairy and protein foods throughout the week.

Milk, cheese, eggs, peanut butter, yogurt, and lean meats are good sources of protein. Bread, oatmeal, grits, rice, cereal, and pancakes provide carbohydrates. Fruits and vegetables are loaded with vitamins and minerals. Choose fruits and vegetables in a variety of colors: yellow, green, red, white, purple, orange, and more!

All foods contain nutrients, but some foods are healthier than others. For example, a potato provides carbohydrates, fiber, and vitamin C plus small amounts of other nutrients. Potato chips, however, may also be loaded with more sugar, salt, and fat than the body needs. Most children do not eat large amounts of food, so provide foods that are nutritious.

TRYING NEW FOODS

Food preferences are learned. Your child may dislike a food at one time but then like that food several weeks later, or vice versa. Try to get a new food on your child's tongue at least eighteen times, even for just a tiny taste of the food. Start with one or two bites of a new food. If your child does not like it, try it again another day.

Try preparing and offering foods in various ways. For example, vegetables can be served lightly steamed, raw with dip, and as part of other foods, such as soups.

Children have more taste buds than adults and are therefore more sensitive to flavors. Foods with pepper or other spices may taste too hot or spicy for your child. Do not insist that your child eat or finish a food. By letting your child stop eating when she or he is full, you are helping to develop good eating habits.

From *Fitness and Nutrition* by Connie Jo Smith, Charlotte M. Hendricks, and Becky S. Bennett, © 2014. Published by Redleaf Press, www.redleafpress.org. This page may be reproduced for classroom use only.

FAMILY ACTIVITY

Cut out the following foods, and assist your child in sorting them into food groups, shapes that are alike, favorite tastes, and so on. First, discuss which foods in this activity you and your child have each tried and which foods you might like to try. Next discuss other foods you each would like to try and in which food groups they belong.

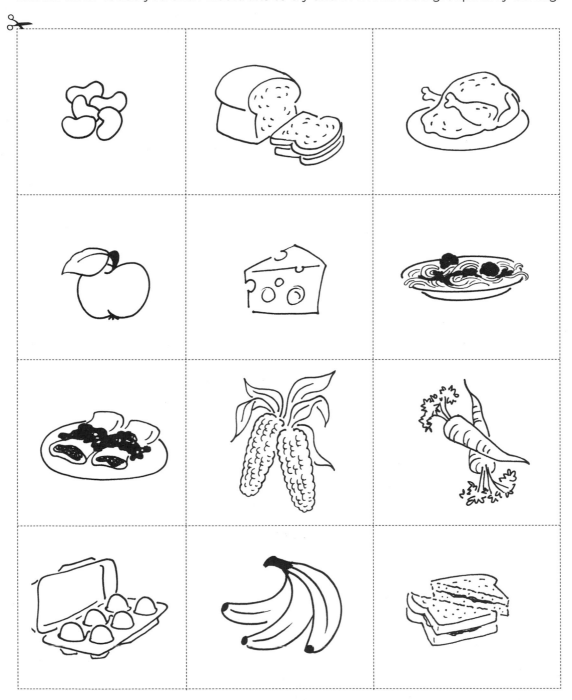

From *Fitness and Nutrition* by Connie Jo Smith, Charlotte M. Hendricks, and Becky S. Bennett, © 2014. Published by Redleaf Press, www.redleafpress.org. This page may be reproduced for classroom use only.

I Share Food, Not Germs!

LEARNING OBJECTIVES

- Children will appropriately pass and serve food (for example, family-style).
- Children will state that germs can be spread by their hands and through food and beverages.
- Children will demonstrate proper ways to share food (for example, by dividing food before beginning to eat or drink).

Illnesses and diseases can spread among children and adults in many ways. Potentially harmful germs, bacteria, and viruses travel on food, beverages, and utensils. Anyone eating or handling these contaminated products may contract an illness or disease.

Illnesses such as colds and influenza are easily and quickly spread among children and adults. Germs can be spread when someone drinks from a glass or straw after an infected person used it. Some diseases spread through the fecal–oral route. Germs may get on a child's hands during toileting; the unclean hands might then contaminate serving utensils or bowls, allowing germs to contaminate another child's hands and enter his mouth when eating.

Some germs, such as staph and salmonella, can contaminate food. If food is not properly prepared and stored, these germs can multiply rapidly, causing severe stomach distress, vomiting, and diarrhea in those who eat the food.

To reduce the potential for infection, both children and adults should wash their hands thoroughly before and after preparing and eating food at mealtime and snacktime and before and after classroom cooking activities.

Family-style meal service and the self-serving of portions are desirable practices for young children. Assist children as they learn to pass serving bowls of food, and supervise them closely as they develop the skills needed to handle serving utensils.

Teach children that eating utensils (forks and spoons) are for individual use; they should not put their utensils in a serving bowl. Provide individual cups or reusable water bottles for drinking, and help children pour water for themselves throughout the day. Be sure to clean and sanitize water bottles each day.

Mealtime and snacktime activities provide opportunities to show children how to share food appropriately. Show children how to cut a sandwich in half before taking a bite, how to pour beverages from a small pitcher into individual cups, and how to use tongs or a napkin to remove a cracker or cookie from a serving tray.

VOCABULARY

before	cut	half	sip
bowl	divide	pass	third
buffet	fountain	pitcher	tongs
canteen	fourth	plate	touch
clean	germ	pour	tray
cup	glass	share	utensil

CREATING THE ENVIRONMENT

- Encourage children to thoroughly wash their hands before eating or handling food. In some facilities, children wash their hands in one room and eat meals in another. If contamination is likely between hand washing and eating, assist children in also using liquid hand sanitizer before eating.

- Prepare food for children just before meal- or snacktime, and serve the food immediately. Leftovers should not remain at room temperature for more than thirty minutes and should be covered and stored in a refrigerator. Contact the local health department for information on cleaning food utensils and proper food preparation and storage.

- Be prepared to address issues regarding food sharing: whether children are allowed to bring food from home and, if so, what measures are in place to ensure proper nutrition and to meet additional storage requirements; whether children are allowed to share food with other children; and what policies need to be set for food adults provide for the classroom on special occasions.

- For cooking activities, the ideal environment includes a refrigerator, paper towels, enough outlets for various appliances, and a sink that is easy to access. If the prepared food will be shared with others, provide serving utensils and small bowls for serving and passing the food. Children may assist in food preparation in many ways, including washing fruits and vegetables and helping to measure ingredients (for example, children can look at the mark on a clear measuring cup or select the correct size spoon). Other activities include stirring, pouring, and reading the recipe together. Adults who handle food that may be consumed should wear food-service gloves to prevent contamination.

■ To further prevent disease transmission, give each child her own food and supplies when classroom cooking activities require handling food with hands and fingers.

EVALUATION

■ Do children pass food to others when requested?

■ Do children use serving utensils appropriately (based on their ability)?

■ Do children talk about ways to share food, not germs?

■ During role playing, do children share food appropriately?

■ Do children wash their hands before eating or preparing food with increasing regularity and fewer reminders?

CHILDREN'S ACTIVITIES

Cups for Everyone

Fill pouring containers with water, adding ice to some of them. Give children individual cups, and explain that they can get drinks with their own cups any time they are thirsty. Provide art supplies, and help each child, as needed, to write his name on his cup. Encourage children to decorate their cups too. Children who do not recognize their names may remember their drawings. Once cups are labeled and decorated, invite children to pour themselves a drink. Stress that they are to wash their hands before pouring and that they should use only their own cups. Children can help one another pour, but they should not share their cups for drinking. Explain briefly that if they drink out of another child's cup, they are sharing germs in addition to water. Identify a place to store cups, and assist each child in placing her cup so that it does not touch other cups when they are being stored. Periodically ask children if they are thirsty and want to get a drink of water.

MATERIALS
- a variety of pouring containers (such as pitchers, empty and clean milk jugs, canteens, and water bottles), water, ice, cups that can be decorated, and art supplies

OTHER IDEAS
- Let children cut or tear out photographs of people drinking water from old catalogs and magazines, and then assist them, as needed, in gluing photos on a group collage. Point out that each person in the photos has his own cup, glass, or bottle for drinking.

- Provide a variety of water bottles, and encourage children to take off the lids and put them back on again to learn how they work.

- Visit a sports store to see all kinds of water bottles and to learn which bottles are used for which sports.

- Take a walk through the program building or visit public places to see a variety of drinking fountains. Explore how each one works. Show children how to drink from the fountain without placing their mouths on it.

Pass the Peas, Please

Invite a small group of children to role-play sharing a meal with you. Instruct children to wash their hands with water and soap and to dry them completely with paper towels. Provide a variety of serving containers with items representing food inside, serving utensils, and a place setting for each child. Include pretend food so children can practice removing it with various utensils. Explain to children that the food is for all of them to share. Ask them to explain how they can share the food without touching the food. Have children identify their own dishes and utensils and then the ones that will be used by the entire group. Reinforce that their individual utensils should not go into containers used by the group and that the group utensils are for serving food and not for eating. Ask the children to pass several dishes, and let them practice passing the containers. Model saying, "Thank you," when dishes are passed to you. Encourage children to politely request that foods be passed to them by other children. After children practice passing, instruct them to use the serving utensils to put pretend food on their plates. Explain that using serving utensils is a way to share food but not germs. After a time, thank the children for coming to dinner, and help them transition to the next activity.

MATERIALS

■ a variety of filled serving containers and utensils (such as a plastic serving bowl with large jingle bells inside and a tablespoon, a wooden bowl with scraps of wadded paper inside and a wooden spoon, a deep metal bowl half filled with water and a ladle, a glass bowl with pinecones inside and a serving spoon, a plastic plate with clay balls on it and tongs, a plastic plate with sponges on it and a serving spatula, a basket containing small blocks and a serving spoon) and place settings of a plate, a fork, and a spoon for each child

OTHER IDEAS

■ Have a pretend tea party with a small group of children, and practice passing pretend sugar and cream.

■ Play "The Sharing Song" by Raffi or Jack Johnson and Friends, and encourage children to sing along.

■ Play passing games, such as Hot Potato or Pass the Parcel. Modify games to allow all children to continue to practice passing throughout the game without any child losing.

- Add serving utensils to the dramatic play interest area so children can practice using them correctly when role-playing. Utensils, like tongs, may also be placed in the table toys interest area so children can practice transferring objects from one container to another.

Buffet Bound

Arrange for children to visit a child-friendly restaurant that has a buffet. Encourage children to observe and discuss the workers and customers. If possible during the visit, go on a kitchen tour to see the food preparation and related containers and utensils. Arrange for a restaurant staff member to explain and show how the cold food is kept cold and the hot food is kept hot. Ask a restaurant staff member to provide a brief review of the rules about eating from the buffet table. Let children eat, and have them practice following the rules. Point out that everyone in the restaurant is sharing food on the buffet without sharing germs. Assist children in making a large group-illustrated thank-you note, and send it to the restaurant staff.

MATERIALS
- chart paper and art supplies

OTHER IDEAS

- Set up a buffet for lunch at the program, and review the rules for sharing food and not germs.

- Invite family members or others who work in a buffet-style restaurant to talk about the rules for diners. Encourage the children to ask questions.

- Invite someone from the health department to talk briefly about restaurant food inspections and to show any tools (such as a thermometer) or paperwork used in the process.

- Find photographs of buffets set with food. Buffet photos may come from online image sites or magazines, or they may be taken at a restaurant. Mount and display the photographs in the classroom, glue the photographs to cardboard and cut the cardboard into puzzle pieces, or glue the photographs onto heavy stock paper to make books.

Half a Cookie

Hold up two puppets. Have one puppet hold a paper cookie that has a bite taken out of it. Introduce the puppet holding the cookie as Jama and the other one as Omar. Put on a short puppet show focusing on Omar asking for some of the cookie and Jama saying he has already taken a bite. Ask children what they think about sharing a cookie with a bite already taken out of it. Explain that if Jama has a cold and takes a bite of a cookie, and then Omar takes a bite of the same cookie, Omar will probably get a cold too. Remind children that germs can be spread by sharing drinks and bites of food that someone else has already tasted. Ask how Omar and Jama might share the food but not germs. Tell children that if they want to share food, it should be divided before anyone takes a bite. Cut a second paper cookie in two, and put half by Omar and half by Jama to show the children how to share.

MATERIALS

- two puppets, two paper cookies, and scissors

OTHER IDEAS

- Provide children with playdough and plastic knives, and have them practice cutting the playdough into halves, thirds, and fourths that can be shared.

- After children have washed their hands, provide bread and table knives or plastic knives so they can practice cutting and sharing bread.

- Read *Give Me Half!* by Stuart J. Murphy.

- Show and discuss the video clip "Ernie Shares Bert's Cookie" on the Sesame Street website at www .sesamestreet.org/video_player /-/pgpv/videoplayer/0/8227e95b -1555-11dd-8211-118eeoe6e3e7/ernie _shares_bert_s_cookie.

Sharing Snacks

In small groups, help children plan and prepare a snack to be shared. Provide a children's cookbook or recipe cards with pictures for them to review for ideas. Ask questions to guide children in selecting food, buying ingredients, fixing food, and appropriately serving and sharing the food without spreading germs. Assist them in determining the amount of food needed to serve all the children. Arrange a trip to the grocery store to purchase food, and assist the children in preparing and serving the food as needed. Help them clean up after preparing and eating the snack.

MATERIALS

- paper, pencils, a children's cookbook or illustrated recipe cards, ingredients (to be identified by the children), and cooking utensils and dishes (to be identified by the children)

OTHER IDEAS

- Involve all children in preparing a snack, and invite another group of children, family members, or program administrators to enjoy and share the snack. Remind children often about sharing food and not germs.

- Add pretend food to the dramatic play interest area so children can practice dividing and sharing food during role playing.

- Provide a few foods (such as an apple, a slice of bread, a bottle of water, a box of raisins, and so on) and have a small group of children evaluate the foods and decide the best way to share them without sharing germs. Once they identify an acceptable way to share food and not germs and after they wash their hands, allow them to share the foods appropriately.

- Read and discuss *Piglet's Picnic: A Story about Food and Counting* by Jessica Souhami.

Something from Everyone

Ask children to wash their hands before story time. Read and discuss *Stone Soup* by Marcia Brown, or any version of the story available. As you read the book, offer a taste of each raw vegetable contributed by a villager for the soup in the story (such as cabbage, carrots, onions, potatoes, mushrooms, and so on). Follow the reading with a discussion of the book, and direct children to wash their hands again before they assist you in preparing vegetables to add to a soup pot for the group to share. Take photos of children preparing the vegetables and eating the finished soup. Once the soup is finished, discuss the differences in how each vegetable tasted raw and cooked. Remind children that the soup was possible because each of them helped to prepare the ingredients. Provide the photos for them to enjoy as they revisit the experience of preparing soup together.

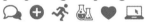

❗ Safety Note: Check and follow your state licensing regulations regarding cooking with children. This experience can be fun and educational even if the soup must be cooked in a kitchen away from the children and the finished product has to be provided to the children to eat. Supervise children closely during any cutting activities.

MATERIALS

■ A copy of *Stone Soup* by Marcia Brown, a variety of vegetables, knives or a food chopper, a pot, water or broth, seasonings (if desired), and a camera

OTHER IDEAS

■ Invite children to look at the photos you took as they prepared and ate stone soup. Help them write a group story about the experience. Compile the photos and dictated sentences from children into a book.

■ Add a few large stones to the dramatic play interest area so children can make stone soup during role playing.

■ Encourage children to find and bring to a central location all toys, puzzles, pictures, and other objects that are related to the story *Stone Soup*. Examples may include a puzzle of a carrot from the table toy interest area, a plastic potato and cooking pot from the dramatic play interest area, and stones from the science and math interest area.

- Use stones to make the shape of letters, write children's names, outline shapes and objects, play hopscotch, count, sort, and engage in many other creative activities.

FAMILY INFORMATION

I SHARE FOOD, NOT GERMS!

It is great when children share toys or crackers, but not when they share germs! Germs that cause diseases can travel in food and beverages and on eating utensils. Colds, influenza, and other illnesses can quickly spread among children who share glasses, cups, or eating utensils.

Sharing a bite of a sandwich or a sip of juice can also spread germs. Children should not eat or drink from the same containers as anyone else, including family members.

HEALTHFUL WAYS TO SHARE

Help children learn healthful ways to share food by demonstrating these practices:

- To share a sandwich or an apple, cut the food before taking a bite.

- To share juice, pour it from the container into the number of glasses needed.

- Use tongs or serving spoons in food dishes. Do not use a spoon you have had in your mouth.

- When taking food from a platter with your hands, take the first item that you touch.

- Use a napkin to take a cookie from a plate.

- Wash your hands before sharing or eating food or drinks.

WHAT NOT TO SHARE

Help your child look around your home for items that should not be shared, such as a toothbrush, a drinking cup, or a partially eaten cookie.

From *Fitness and Nutrition* by Connie Jo Smith, Charlotte M. Hendricks, and Becky S. Bennett, © 2014. Published by Redleaf Press, www.redleafpress.org. This page may be reproduced for classroom use only.

FAMILY ACTIVITY

Glue this picture to one side of an empty cereal box, and then cut out the puzzle pieces, using the lines as guides. After assisting your child to complete the puzzle, discuss how each person in the picture is about to eat and drink, what utensils they are using, and how they might pass the food they are eating to enjoy the meal together without sharing germs.

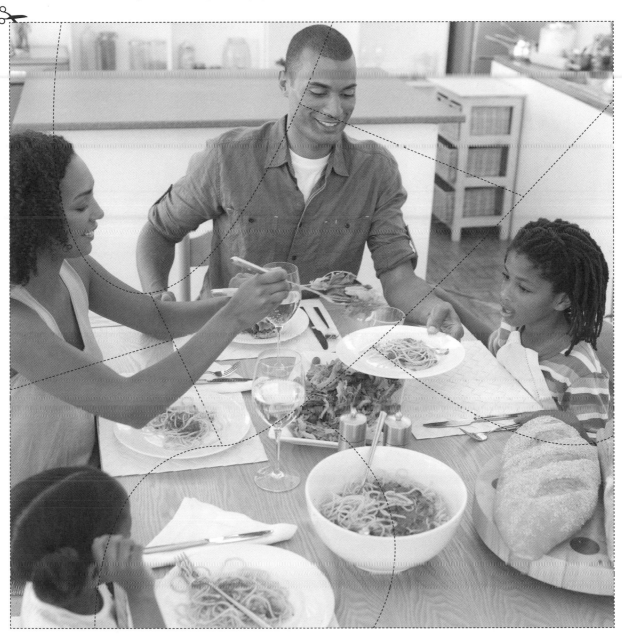

From *Fitness and Nutrition* by Connie Jo Smith, Charlotte M. Hendricks, and Becky S. Bennett, © 2014.
Published by Redleaf Press, www.redleafpress.org. This page may be reproduced for classroom use only.